PUBLIC HEALTH: PRACTICES, METHODS AND POLICIES

ARBOVIRUS

PUBLIC HEALTH EXPERIENCE FROM ZAMBIA

PUBLIC HEALTH: PRACTICES, METHODS AND POLICIES

Additional books in this series can be found on Nova's website under the Series tab.

Additional e-books in this series can be found on Nova's website under the e-book tab.

PUBLIC HEALTH: PRACTICES, METHODS AND POLICIES

ARBOVIRUS

PUBLIC HEALTH EXPERIENCE FROM ZAMBIA

SETER SIZIYA
MAZYANGA L. MAZABA
AND
JOAV MERRICK
EDITORS

nova publishers
New York

Library of Congress Cataloging-in-Publication Data

ISBN: 978-1-63463-601-8

Library of Congress Control Number: 2014956461

Published by Nova Science Publishers, Inc. † New York

CONTENTS

INTRODUCTION

In: Arbovirus
Editors: S. Siziya, M. L. Mazaba et al.
ISBN: 978-1-63463-601-8

Chapter 1

INTRODUCTION: PUBLIC HEALTH AND ARBOVIRAL DISEASES

***Seter Siziya, BA(Ed), MSc, PhD**[*1,2], **Mazyanga L Mazaba, BSc, MSc**[3,4], **and Joav Merrick, MD, MMedSc, DMSc**[5-9]*

[1]School of Medicine, Copperbelt University, Ndola, Zambia
[2]University of Lusaka, Lusaka, Zambia, [3]World Health Organization, Lusaka, Zambia
[4]University Teaching Hospital, Ministry of Health, Lusaka, Zambia
[5]National Institute of Child Health and Human Development, Jerusalem
[6]Office of the Medical Director, Health Services, Division for Intellectual and Developmental Disabilities, Ministry of Social Affairs and Social Services, Jerusalem
[7]Division of Pediatrics, Hadassah Hebrew University Medical Center, Mt Scopus Campus, Jerusalem, Israel
[8]Kentucky Children's Hospital, University of Kentucky College of Medicine, Lexington, Kentucky, United States of America
[9]Center for Healthy Development, School of Public Health, Georgia State University, Atlanta, United States of America

[*] Correspondence: Professor Seter Siziya, Department of Clinical Sciences, School of Medicine, Copperbelt University, POBox 71191, Ndola, Zambia. E-mail: ssiziya@gmail.com.

Introduction

Arboviruses have become significant causes of public health problems with potential for epidemics and unprecedented spread (1, 2). Large epidemics have occurred and will continue to occur, unless we remain extremely vigilant, respond promptly, and have more to offer than isolation and quarantine (3). Arboviral diseases include: West Nile virus disease, Yellow fever and dengue among others (4). These viruses have caused wide-spread morbidity in sub-Saharan Africa and worldwide (5). The changing epidemiology of arboviruses, the changing virulence of arboviruses, increased vector population responsible for transmission of diseases, the growing population sizes and rapid urbanization cause changes in equilibrium of vectors and hosts, thus, increasing chances of outbreaks and epidemics (6) and therefore a constant watch on the pattern of arboviral diseases through surveillance is inevitable.

Surveillance

Public health surveillance which is the ongoing systematic collection, analysis, interpretation, and dissemination of health data (7) can serve as an early warning system for impending epidemics (8). The objectives of a public health surveillance system are to detect epidemics; to guide immediate action; to measure the burden of disease; to monitor trends; to evaluate public policy; to detect changes in health practices and their effects; to describe the clinical course of disease; to guide the planning, implementation and evaluation of program and to prioritize the allocation of health resources (9). There are two types of surveillance: Passive and active surveillance.

Passive disease surveillance refers to the receipt of reports of disease from health staff that are required by law to submit such reports without being reminded to do so and forms may be collected from health facilities. Data from passive surveillance is often incomplete partly because there are no incentives for health staff to complete the forms. Active disease surveillance refers to contacting health staff that is provided with feedback or other incentives to search for cases and as a result data is more complete than that from passive surveillance. This type of surveillance is usually seasonal to coincide with periods of high disease frequency and generally yields a much higher percentage of actual cases as compared to passive surveillance. Active surveillance is used also during outbreaks to identify additional cases (10, 11).

Active surveillance of population movements can provide data for planning emergency interventions and for general disease surveillance (12).

Characteristics of well-conducted surveillance include: acceptability, flexibility, high predictive value positive, quality, representativeness, sensitivity, simplicity, stability, timeliness and validity (13) and among these, the following characteristics are more important in surveillance detecting outbreaks of diseases: Timeliness, stability, representativeness, flexibility (14) and validity. To validate the suspicions of the findings during surveillance, confirmed diagnosis through laboratory testing is a necessity. The laboratory plays a key role in providing information that can be used to target and focus resources containment and possible eradication of diseases (15).

A number of epidemics caused by arboviruses have been documented over the centuries (16-20), and surveillance has played an important role in these milestones (21). The fact that arbovirus epidemics continue to occur, it suggests that public health surveillance is either nonexistence or has failed to detect impending epidemics. In resource constrained countries for structured surveillance, it has been suggested that emphasis should be placed on detecting alerts from formal (health facilities) or informal sources (community informants) rather than on analysis of surveillance data, which often is incomplete and has low timeliness (22).

Brucner and Checchi (23) concluded in a systematic review that timeliness of detection, investigation and response was poor for most outbreaks that occurred in 22 of the resource constrained countries, thus making containment of the epidemics extremely difficulty. Public health surveillance system should be frequently evaluated so that it is made to be the best strategy to avert epidemics.

REFERENCES

[1] Gubler DJ. The global emergence/resurgence of arboviral diseases as public health problems. Arch Med Res 2002;33:330–422.

[2] Weaver SC, Reisen WK. Present and future arboviral threats. Antiviral Res 2010;85:328–45.

[3] Piot P, Muyembe JJ, Edmunds WJ. Ebola in west Africa: from disease outbreak to humanitarian crisis. Lancet Infect Dis 2014. Pii S1473-3099(14)70956-9.

[4] Gould EA, Higgs S, Buckley A, Gritsun TS. Potential Arbovirus Emergence and Implications for the United Kingdom. Emerg Infect Dis 2006;12:549–55.

[5] Dash AP, Bhatia R, Sunyoto T, Mourya DT. Emerging and re-emerging arboviral diseases in Southeast Asia. J Vector Borne Dis 2013;50:77–84.

[6] Abdalla S, Panjabi R. Control of communicable disease. In: The John Hopkins and Red Cross Red Crescent. Public health guide in emergencies, 2nd edition. Geneva: International Federation of Red Cross and Red Crescent Societies, 2008:285-371.

[7] Thacker SB, Choi K, Brachman PS. The surveillance of infectious diseases. JAMA 1983;249:1181-5.

[8] WHO. Public health surveillance. Accessed 18 October 2014. URL: http://www.who.int/topics/public_health_surveillance/en/

[9] German RR, Lee LM, Horan JM, Milstein RL, Pertowski CA, Waller MN, Guidelines Working Group Centers for Disease Control and Prevention (CDC). Updated guidelines for evaluating public health surveillance systems: recommendations from the Guidelines Working Group. MMWR Recomm Rep 2001;50(RR-13):1-35.

[10] Manitoba Health, Public Health. Communicable Disease Surveillance. Communicable Disease Management Protocol Manual. Accessed 18 October 2014. URL: http://www.gov.mb.ca/health/publichealth/cdc/protocol/surveillance.pdf.

[11] London School of Hygiene and Tropical Medicine. The use of epidemiological tools in conflict-affected populations: open-access educational resources for policy-makers. Accessed 18 October 2014. URL: http://conflict.lshtm.ac.uk/page_75.htm.

[12] World Health Organisation. Control of communicable diseases and prevention of epidemics. Accessed 19 October 2014. URL: http://www.who.int/water_sanitation_health/hygiene/emergencies/em2002chap11.pdf.

[13] US Department of Health and Human Services, CDC. Principles of epidemiology in public health practice: An introduction to applied epidemiology and biostatistics, 3rd ed. Accessed 19 October 2014. URL: https://www.scribd.com/doc/116813789/Principles-of-Epidemiology-in-Public-Health-Practice.

[14] Sosin DM, Hopkins RS. Monitoring disease and risk factors: surveillance. In: Pencheon D, Melzer D, Gray M, Guest C, eds. Oxford handbook of public health, 2nd ed. Oxford: Oxford University Press, 2006.

[15] IVB. Polio laboratory manual, 4th ed. Geneva: World Health Organization, 2004. Accessed 2014 October 21. URL: http://whqlibdoc.who.int/hq/2004 /WHO_IVB_04.10.pdf.

[16] Gubler DJ. Dengue and dengue hemorrhagic fever. Clin Microbiol Rev 1998;11:480–96.

[17] Henchal EA, Putnak JR. The dengue viruses. Clin Microbiol Rev 1990;3:376–96.

[18] Smithburn KC, Hughes TP, Burke AW, Paul JH. A Neurotropic virus isolated from the blood of a native of Uganda. Am J Trop Med 1940;20:471–92.

[19] Whitehorn J, Farrar J. Dengue. Br Med Bull 2010;95:161–73.

[20] Guzman MG, Halstead SB, Artsob H, Buchy P, Farrar J, Gubler DJ, Hunsperger E, Kroeger A, Margolis HS, Martinez E, Nathan MB, Pelegrino JL, et al. Dengue: A continuing global threat. Nat Rev Microbiol 2010;8(Suppl 12):S7–16.

[21] Hanley KA, Weaver SC. Arbovirus evolution. In: Domingo E, Parrish CR, Holland JJ, eds. Origin and evolution of viruses, 2nd ed. London: Elsevier, 2008:351-87.

[22] Anonymous. Early warning surveillance and response in emergencies: WHO technical workshop, December 2009. Wkly Epidemiol Rec 2010;85:129-36.
[23] Bruckner C, Checchi F. Detection of infectious disease outbreaks in twenty-two fragile states, 2000-2010: a systematic review. Confl Health 2011;5:13.

SECTION ONE: ARBOVIRUSES IN ZAMBIA

In: Arbovirus ISBN: 978-1-63463-601-8
Editors: S. Siziya, M. L. Mazaba et al.

Chapter 2

ARBOVIRUSES IN NORTH-WESTERN AND WESTERN PROVINCES OF ZAMBIA

***Mazyanga L Mazaba, BSc, MSc*[*1,2], Olusegun Babaniyi, MBBS, MPH, MSc[1], Freddie Masaninga, BSc, MSc, PhD[1], Peter Songolo, MBChB, MPH[1], Idah Mweene-Ndumba, BSc, MPH[1,2], and Seter Siziya, BA(Ed), MSc, PhD[3,4]**

[1]World Health Organization, Lusaka, Zambia
[2]University Teaching Hospital, Lusaka, Zambia
[3]School of Medicine, Copperbelt University, Ndola, Zambia
[4]University of Lusaka, Lusaka, Zambia

Arboviruses have caused wide-spread morbidity in sub-Saharan Africa and worldwide. The objective was to present a synthesis of the findings on arboviruses infections determined from a 2013 yellow fever risk assessment survey conducted in North-Western and Western provinces of Zambia. We reviewed published and unpublished papers on prevalence and correlates for arboviruses. Prevalence rates for arboviruses infections were 10.3% for West Nile, 6.0% for Zika, 4.1% for dengue, 0.5% for yellow fever and 11.5% for any arbovirus infection. Persons aged less than 5 years were 63% less likely to have infection compared to persons

[*] Correspondence: Mazyanga L Mazaba, EPI Unit, World Health Organization, Lusaka, Zambia and Virology Unit, University Teaching Hospital, Lusaka, Zambia. E-mail: mazmazli@yahoo.com.

aged 45 years or older. In-door residual spraying was associated with reduced risk for West Nile or Zika viruses infections. Visiting Angola was significantly associated with increased risk for dengue, West Nile and Zika arboviruses infections. Respondents living in grass roofed houses were 2-3 times more likely to have any of the infections compared to those living in houses with asbestos roofs. A total of 1401 adult mosquitoes were collected comprising 28.9% Aedes, 37.0% Anopheles, 471 (33.6%) Culex and 71 (5.1%) Mansonia. The factors: roof type and visiting Angola in addition to arbovirus-specific infection correlates should be considered in developing interventions to control them in North-Western and Western provinces of Zambia.

INTRODUCTION

Recently the following arboviruses were identified in Zambia: Yellow fever (1), dengue (2), West Nile (Mweene-Ndumba et al., unpublished) and Zika (Babaniyi et al., unpublished). These viruses, all among the group B of arboviruses under the genus Flavivirus, have caused wide-spread morbidity in sub-Saharan Africa and worldwide (3).

Yellow fever

Yellow fever known to occur commonly in certain parts of Africa and South America but absent in Asia (4) is caused by yellow fever virus. It is unclear why yellow fever does not occur in Asia. The typical symptoms in yellow fever infected persons include fever, muscle pains, headache, nausea and vomiting from the third to sixth day of infection. Although up-to 85% of illnesses resolve at this stage, others progress to a severe disease following a brief 2-24 hour remission of symptoms. The symptoms in severe disease include nausea, vomiting, epigastric pain, renal failure, jaundice and haemorrhaging. At this stage of the disease about half of patients die within 10–14 days, and those who survive develop immunity for the rest of their lives (5). There is no cure for yellow fever (6). However, there is an effective vaccine for the prevention of yellow fever (7). About 200 000 people are infected with yellow fever annually in the tropics of Africa and South America (4) and causes about 30 000 deaths each year (8).

Dengue

Dengue virus is the cause of dengue disease. The World Health Organization documents existence of 4 serotypes of dengue virus. Infection by one serotype allows lifelong immunity to only the specific infecting serotype. Re-infection with another serotype can occur and lead to dengue haemorrhagic fever (9). Although, dengue virus infection is often unapparent (10), signs and symptoms for dengue virus infection vary from mild, non-specific symptoms to classic dengue fever, with high fevers and severe arthralgia. The non-specific symptoms include fever, nausea/vomiting, rash, aches and pains, abdominal pain or tenderness, persistent vomiting, clinical fluid accumulation, mucosal bleed, lethargy/restlessness, liver enlargement of 2 cm or more and increase in HCT concurrent with rapid decrease in platelet count. Symptoms associated with severe dengue include severe plasma leakage leading to dengue shock syndrome, fluid accumulation with respiratory distress, bleeding and organ (such as liver, Central Nervous System and heart) involvement (11). About 1–5% of the patients will die if not adequately attended to and less than 1% of the patients will die if adequately clinically managed (12). However, 26% of the severely ill patients will die (13). There is no cure for dengue fever. However, symptomatic treatment can reduce mortality from DHF to less than 1% (14). Dengue vaccine is not available for use (15), although a vaccine trial is underway (16). Dengue disease is globally distributed in both endemic and epidemic transmission cycles. Bhatt et al. (17) estimated that of the 96 million dengue infections globally in 2010, 70% of them were from Asia, 14% from the Americas and 16% from Africa (18-20).

West Nile virus

About 20% of the people who become infected with West Nile virus do not develop any symptoms (21). Those who develop symptoms will have headache, body aches, joint pains, vomiting, diarrhoea and rash. Most people with this type of West Nile virus disease recover completely, but fatigue and weakness can last for weeks or months. In its severe form, patients will develop a serious neurologic illness whose symptoms include headache, high fever, neck stiffness, disorientation, coma, tremors, seizures or paralysis. About 10% of people who develop neurologic infection will die (22). There is no treatment or vaccine for West Nile virus infection (23). However, vaccine development is underway (24). West Nile virus infection is the most wide spread flavivirus, covering Africa, Europe, Asia, Australia (Kunjin), North and South America (25).

Zika

The symptoms for Zika virus infection that were based on a limited number of case reports and outbreak investigations (26,27) are acute onset of fever, non-purulent conjunctivitis, headache, arthralgia, myalgia, asthenia, rash (in general maculo-papular) and, less frequently, retro-orbital pain, anorexia, vomiting, diarrhoea and abdominal pain. In the literature, Zika is described as a mild, self-limiting febrile illness lasting 28 days without severe complications, no fatalities and a low hospitalisation rate (28, 29). In a well investigated, 2007 Zika virus infection outbreak on Yap Island in the Federated States of Micronesia (29) the common symptoms were rash, fever, arthralgia and conjunctivitis. The other symptoms were included myalgia, headache and retro-orbital pain. There is no specific anti-viral treatment for Zika virus infection and there is no vaccine (26). Zika virus infection has been reported in Africa (Nigeria, Sierra Leone, Ivory Coast, Cameroon, Senegal, Central Africa Republic, Uganda (26) and Kenya (30) and in Asia (Malaysia, Pakistan, Cambodia, Thailand, Indonesia, French Polynesia and Federated States of Micronesia (27).

Vectors

The vectors for yellow fever include Aedes africanus (in Africa) or Haemagogus species (in the Americas) (31, 32), Aedes simpsoni and Aedes albopictus (33). Yellow fever virus is primarily transmitted by Aedes (Stegomyia) aegypti and Aedes (Stegomyia) africanus (34). Dengue virus is transmitted between people by mosquito species Aedes aegypti and Aedes albopictus (35). The main vector associated with Dengue virus is Aedes aegypti (36). West Nile virus (WNV) is transmitted through the bites of infective Culex mosquitoes (37-39). Zika virus is spread by the Aedes species of mosquito including the Aedes aegypti mosquito (40). In summary, Aedes aegypti is the main vector for yellow fever, dengue and Zika viruses, while Culex mosquitoes is a vector for West Nile virus.

The objectives for this study is to present a synthesis of the findings from a yellow fever risk assessment in terms of the prevalence rates for the arboviruses and factors associated with the infections.

OUR STUDY

Studies on arboviruses in Zambia were based on a cross sectional survey conducted in 2013 for yellow fever risk assessment.

Study site

Zambia was administratively, divided into ten provinces. Each province was in turn subdivided into districts. Each district was further subdivided into constituencies and wards. For statistical purposes each ward was subdivided into Census Supervisory Areas (CSAs) and these were in turn subdivided into Standard Enumeration Areas (SEAs). The 2008-2010 census mapping exercise in preparation for the 2010 census of population and housing, demarcated the CSAs within wards, wards within constituencies and constituencies within districts. In total, at the time of constructing the 2010 census frame, Zambia had 74 districts, 150 constituencies, 1,421 wards. Wards were further divided into Census Supervisory Areas (CSAs), which were in turn divided into Standard Enumeration Areas (SEAs). The SEAs were also stratified by urban and rural strata. The listing of SEAs had information on number of households and the population. The study sites, North-Western and Western provinces (see figure 1), were conveniently selected being the provinces that were classified as areas of low potential risk of Yellow fever. Western province borders with Angola. Western province had 7 districts with a total of 1,902 SEAs. Fishing was the main occupation in the province. The population of the province was 854,890 (41). Meanwhile, North-Western province had borders with Angola in the west and DR Congo in the north. A total of 1,178 SEAs had been demarcated in North-Western province in the 6 districts of the province. Peasantry farming (mainly cultivating maize, cotton and groundnuts) was the major economic activity in North-Western province. It had a population of 695,599 (41). The study area was divided into three main agro ecological zones (42) that were classified based mainly on the rainfall patterns. Zone I was characterized by low rainfall, short growing season, high temperatures during the growing season, and a high risk of drought. Zone III was characterized by high rainfall, long growing season, low probability of drought, and cooler temperatures during the growing season. Zone II fell in between Zones I and III for most climatic variables. There were great variations in the agro-ecological features (rainfall, elevation, mean temperatures, vegetation and soils) of the three zones and within zones themselves. The location of the ecological zones is shown figure 2. Agro-ecological Zone I covered the Northern part of the country, Zone III was furthest South and Zone II was intermediate between zones I and III. Our study area was covered by Agro-ecological Zones I, IIb and III.

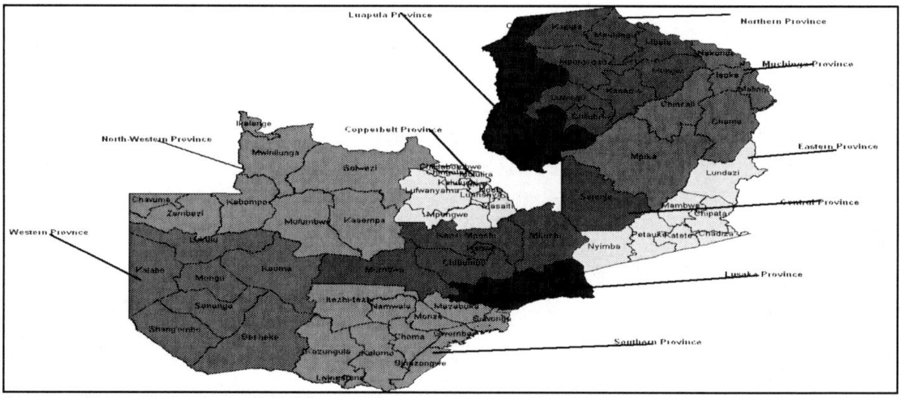

Source: Central Statistical Office (40).

Figure 1. Map of Zambia showing the locations of provinces and districts.

In a demographic health survey, Central Statistical Office et al. (43) reported that 46.9 and 53.2% of the population slept under an insecticide treated net in the previous night to the survey in Western and North-Western Provinces respectively.

Human seroprevalence study

Study population

This assessment was carried out among individuals aged nine months or older located within households sampled in the selected study sites.

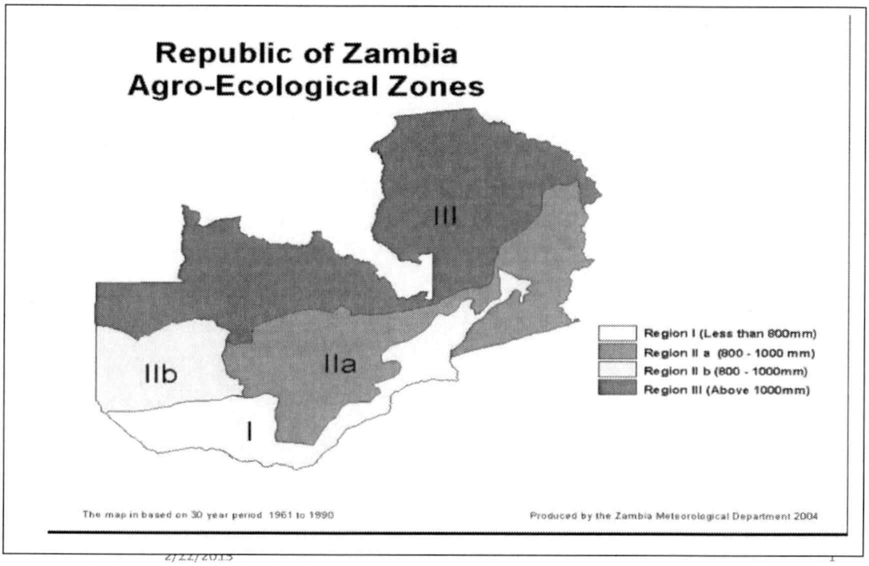

Source: Zambia Meteorological Department (41).

Figure 2. Agro-ecological zones in Zambia.

Sample size, inclusion/exclusion criteria and sampling

Sample size

The sample size calculation was based on the assumption that the seroprevalence was 7% based on the study conducted by Robinson (44). In order to design an efficient study to compare the findings with those obtained in that study, the sample size for the current proposed study was comparable to the sample size done by Robinson (44).

Persons aged 5 years or older

In estimating the sample size for persons aged 5 years or older, the following parameters were considered: a prevalence of 7%, desired precision or confidence interval (d) of $\pm 3\%$, and a design effect (DE) of 2 and an 80% response rate.

$$n_{min} = 2 \times \frac{1.96^2 \times 7 \times (100 - 7)}{3^2}$$

$$= 556$$

and applying the response rate $n_{min} = 556/0.8 = 695$.

Considering sex, we aimed to recruit 700 male and 700 female participants in each province. Assuming an average of 4 persons aged 5 years or older in each household, a total of 12 households in each of the 30 cluster was to be recruited in the survey. The total number of persons that would be recruited from each province was 1,806, totalling 3,612 from both provinces.

Persons under the age of 5 years

The seroprevalence of children was about half that for older children, and in estimating the sample size for persons aged below 5 years, the following parameters were considered: a prevalence of 3.5%, desired precision or confidence interval (d) of ±3.4%, and a design effect (DE) of 2 and an 80% response rate. The total number of persons aged less than 5 years that would be surveyed was computed as follows:

Formula: $n_{min} = DE \times \dfrac{Z^2 \times p \times (1-p)}{d^2}$

where Z = 1.96

$$n_{min} = 2 \times \frac{1.96^2 \times 3.5 \times (100 - 3.5)}{3.4^2}$$

$$= 225$$

and applying the response rate $n_{min} = 225/0.8 = 282$. Therefore, in each province 406 children would be recruited for the survey.

Inclusion/exclusion criteria

Any individual aged 9 months or older and who was a member of a sampled household and resident in the study site for at least seven days. Individuals who received yellow fever vaccination in the last ten years would be eligible to participate in the survey.

Any person, who was either less than 9 months of age, or any person regardless of age, who resided in the study site for a period of less than seven days prior to the survey was excluded from the study. Determining the seroprevalence in children under the age of nine months raises the risk of false positive results as children under this age may still carry maternal antibodies from immunized or exposed mothers.

Sampling

The sample was drawn using a two-stage cluster sampling technique using probability proportional to size. A list of SEAs in each province constituted the sampling frame. The sampling was designed to achieve fairly good estimates at the provincial level of analysis, and not representing the subdivisions of the province.

First stage selection

At the first sampling stage, the sampled SEAs were selected with probability to size (PPS) from the ordered list of SEAs on the census 2010 sampling frame. The measure of size for each SEA was based on the household size identified in the 2010 Census (41). In order to ensure representation from all administrative areas, the frame was sorted by district, constituency, region, CSA and SEA.

Second stage selection

In each selected cluster, the first household that was selected was located in the middle of the cluster. The direction that followed from the middle of the cluster was selected at random. The remaining participants were selected in that direction. If the number of participants was not met, the team got back to the middle of the cluster and selected a direction at random and went in that direction until the required number of participants was surveyed. Figure 3 shows the distribution of the surveyed households.

Study variables

Dependent variables

A case with evidence of yellow fever exposure was defined as any individual aged 9 months or older whose blood sample was confirmed to have yellow fever exposure through any of the following: Detection of yellow fever virus-specific IgG and IgM antibodies with yellow fever virus-specific neutralizing antibodies at least four-fold higher than neutralizing antibodies against other flaviviruses. Yellow fever exposure status was therefore determined by way of laboratory testing as ‘positive’ for a respondent with laboratory evidence of yellow fever exposure or as ‘negative’ for a respondent who did not have laboratory evidence of yellow fever exposure or as “indeterminate” for a respondent with a less than a four-fold difference in titters between yellow fever and other flaviviruses.

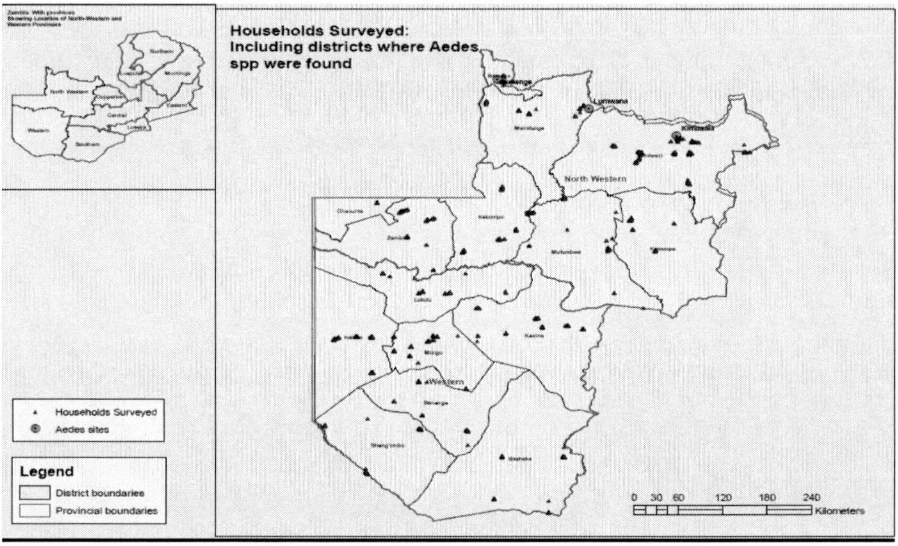

Figure 3. Distribution of surveyed households.

Independent variables

The independent variables included demographic data: age, sex, occupation, history and time of yellow fever vaccination, and use of mosquito preventive measures. For the purposes of the sero-survey, a vaccinated person against yellow fever was defined as a person with a valid yellow fever vaccination certificate.

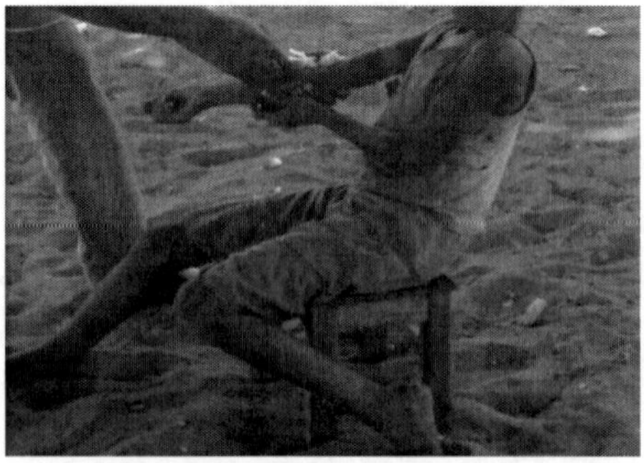

Figure 4. Blood collection from a participant by venepuncture.

Laboratory procedure

Each study participant was assigned a study number and the corresponding blood sample was labeled with the same study number. The study number was linked to the laboratory result and questionnaire. About 3 to 5 millilitres of blood was collected from each participant by venepuncture and collected in an EDTA tube (see figure 4). The samples were transported to a field laboratory on ice, where plasma was separated into labelled cryovials (see figure 5). At the close of the field work, the samples were transported to the University Teaching Hospital Virology Laboratory (UTHVL) for testing.

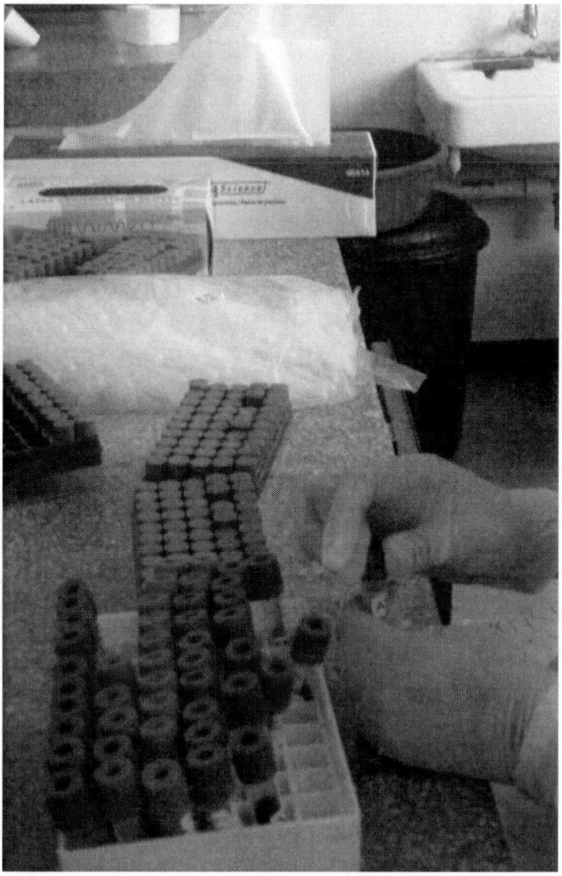

Figure 5. Separation of plasma into labelled cryovials.

Each plasma sample was tested for both yellow fever virus-specific IgG and IgM antibodies by the ELISA method described in the (45) at the UTHVL. All yellow fever virus IgG positive and IgM positive specimens were referred to the Institute Pasteur in Dakar, Senegal which serves as the World Health Organization Africa region reference laboratory for yellow fever. In Dakar, the specimens were subjected to repeat yellow fever virus-specific IgG and IgM Enzyme Linked Immunoassay (ELISA) testing in order to reconfirm the primary results. They were also assessed for IgG and IgM antibodies against other flaviviruses known to cause haemorrhagic fever-like disease including Dengue, Zika and West Nile viruses that are also known to elicit cross-reactivity in antibody ELISA tests. All samples giving a yellow fever virus-specific antibody positive result either in Lusaka or Dakar, were analysed for yellow fever virus neutralising antibodies by Plaque Reduction Neutralisation Testing (PRNT) using standard methods.

Interpretation of laboratory results

Participants with PRNT titres ≥1:10 were considered as being yellow fever seropositive, while those having PRNT titres ≥1:20 were considered to have seroprotective levels of antibodies against yellow fever virus either through natural infection or through vaccination. Those participants who were found to have Immunoglobulin (Ig) M or G antibodies to dengue, West Nile and Zika viruses were considered as having had the respective diseases.

Data collection and quality control

A detailed semi structured questionnaire was used to collect information. The questionnaires were pre-tested to validate the appropriateness of the questions to capture the required information. During the data collection process, questionnaires were checked for inconsistencies and completeness on a daily basis. All data were entered in an Epi-Info data entry screen that had consistency and range checks embedded in it. Further editing was conducted by running frequencies during the analysis stage. Epi data files were exported to SPSS for data analysis.

Data analysis

The data was summarized to describe the occurrence of arboviruses infected individuals in absolute numbers and percentage by place (residence, travel or work) and person (age, sex, occupation). Further analysis was conducted to determine independent factors associated with arboviruses seropositivity. Odds ratios were used to estimate the magnitude of associations.

Ethical considerations in the human seroprevalence study

Ethical clearance was sought from the Tropical Diseases Research Centre Research Ethics Committee, and ethical standards were adhered to throughout this study. Information obtained from the study participants was treated as confidential through the use of anonymous identifiers and restricting the access to collected data only to people directly involved in the study. Respondents were provided with information on possible study risks, for example pain and swelling at the venous-puncture site. In addition information on study benefits like: providing information on yellow fever and its prevention was also provided. Further, the collective benefit of the study of informing the national yellow fever policy was highlighted to the study participants. Informed consent was sought from study participants. Guardians provided assent for the participation of persons under the consenting age. They were asked to read or have read to them, understand and sign/thumbprint an informed consent form. Responsible adults in the household were identified to give proxy consent on behalf of minors. Study participants were informed that their individual test results were not to be relayed to them since the results were not linked to individual participants due to use of unique identifiers and in addition, past exposure to YF carries no future risk.

Socio-mobilisation and community engagement

Before data and specimen collection in any cluster, the community leaders and members were engaged to explain the nature and intention of the study (see figure 6). It was emphasized that participation was voluntary.

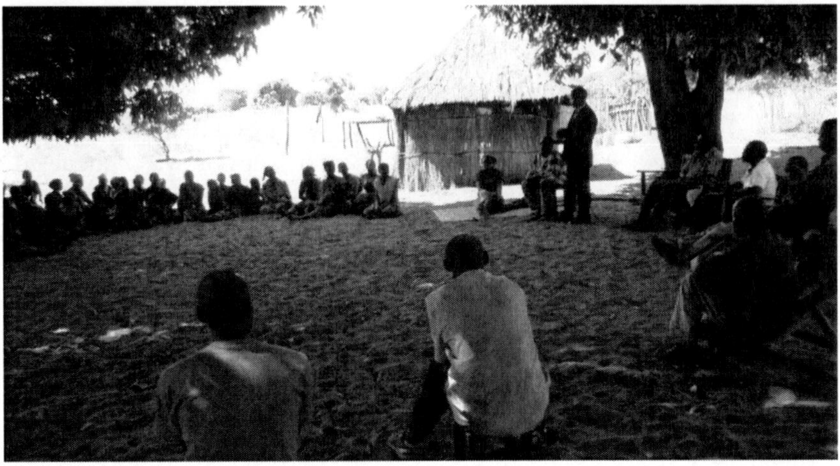

Figure 6. Social mobilization and community engagement.

Mosquitoes study

All three agro-ecological zones were considered for mosquito sampling. Each zone had unique features which affected the types and abundance of mosquitoes present. Attempts were made to collect mosquitoes in all zones with a preference for collecting mosquitoes from at least two distinct areas within each zone. Mosquitoes were identified and sorted in mono-specific batch and, if appropriate, tested for the presence of yellow fever virus by RT-PCR. In addition to sampling adult mosquitoes, larvae was sampled especially in urban centers but also in forested and intermediate areas to the towns, in order to identify more clearly the types of mosquito species in the environment.

Sample size and sampling in the mosquito survey

Attempts were made to collect mosquitoes in all zones since each selected zone contained unique features that could affect types and abundance of mosquitoes present in the area. Eight sampling sites from each province were selected. Adult and larval forms of mosquitoes were sampled in various sites in urban and peri-urban, forest and along plains and on island of the study areas in order to identify the types of mosquito species that occurred in the sampled areas. In order to obtain current information on the level of yellow fever viral circulation in the selected provinces, different sampling techniques were used to sample the mosquito populations. Mosquitoes were sampled around all the 12 selected households in the human survey in each Cluster.

Adult mosquito sampling

Adult mosquitoes were sampled by three groups of researchers (three to four persons per team), who were vaccinated against yellow fever virus and received prior chemoprophylaxis against malaria. Sampling methods that were used were backpack aspirators, aspiration using a mouth aspirator tube, CDC light trap and the Gravid Light traps. Mosquito collections were made inside and outside households.

Indoor adult: Resting mosquitoes were collected by an aspirator (back pack or the use of a mouth aspirator tube) using a torch to locate them. Knockdown spray catch with a pyrethroids insecticide in randomly selected dwellings were also done commencing at 06.00 hours.

Outdoor: Mosquitoes were captured using backpack aspirator; CDC light trap and Gravid light trap for collecting gravid (egg-laying) females to increase the chance for virus isolation. Sampling outdoor with back pack aspirator was done between 16.00 and 19.00 hours.

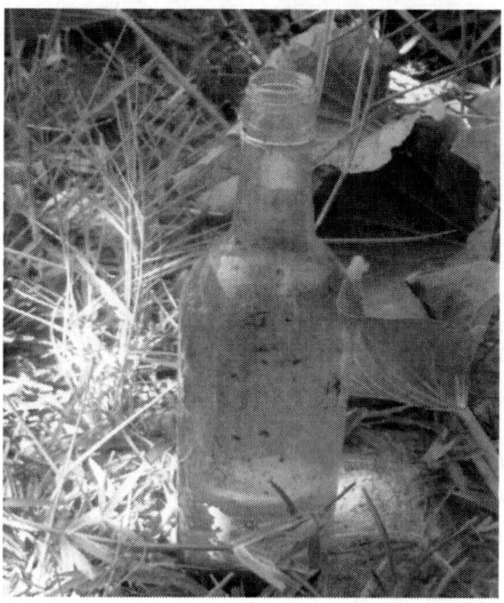

Figure 7. Containers holding water located outside house.

Larvae/pupae sampling

Larval sampling was done in selected premises in each locality visited. Containers holding water located outside (such as the ones displayed in figure 7) and inside households (domestic and peri-domestic) were inspected for larvae/pupae in each cluster visited in order to estimate risk indices.

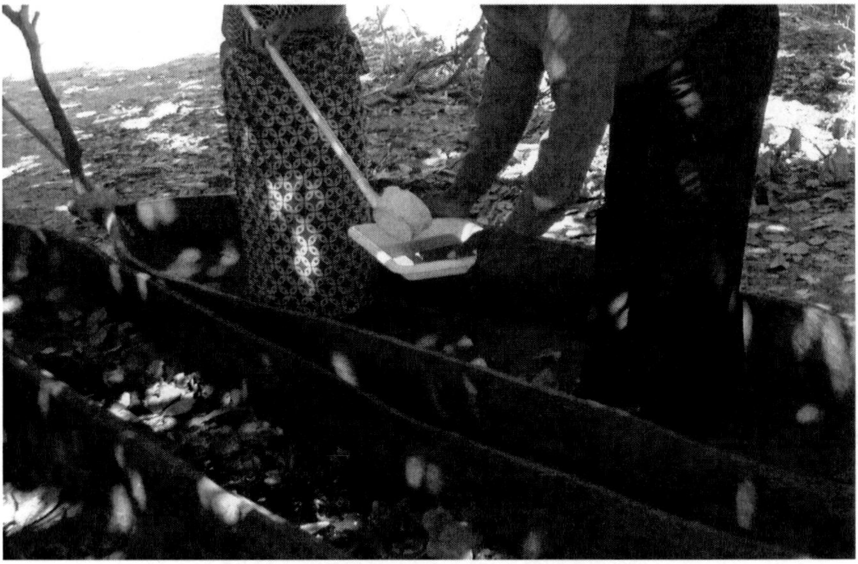

Figure 8. Scooping mosquito larvae from large water bodies onto white trays.

Scoops were used to collect/transfer mosquito larvae from large water bodies onto white trays (see figure 8) from where larvae were pipetted into bottles labelled with information on date, province, cluster name, site of collection in order to identify the source of the larvae. In the domestic environment, artificial and natural mosquito breeding site were inspected.

An attempt was made to count larvae and pupae in each container found positive to estimate absolute population density per habitation unit. Larvae were counted directly for small quantity and estimated using a correlation between the mean number of larvae in deeper and the total volume of the water in the container.

Specific entomological activities conducted in the assessment

Containers with at least one larva or pupa were considered as positive and these larvae were sent to the insectary at the Tropical Diseases Research

Centre for rearing and identification of the emerging adult stages. Samples reared in the insectary allowed an estimation of the population sex ratio and the density of mosquito females in relation to human population density.

The following observations were made: (a) Mosquito species breeding inside/outside houses, (b) The proximity of the houses to potential vector breeding sites i.e., how far the houses were located from forests/woodlands, or any plantations where vectors could be breeding, (c) Eggs of any possible vectors breeding in the vicinity of houses and also in forests/ woodlands/plantations, (d) Adult mosquitoes resting in vegetation around houses and at the periphery of woodlands/forests and in plantations, (e) Adult mosquitoes flying in the evening, dawn and at night in and outside households and in woodlands/forests and (f) Any possible animals that could serve as reservoirs of yellow fever virus.

Investigating viral infection in yellow fever mosquito vectors

Assessment of mosquitoes involved the determination of mosquito species around the selected 12 households per cluster in the same households where human survey was conducted. A record was kept of each mosquito in order to determine overall number of each species captured. Special focus was placed on mosquitoes involved in yellow fever viral transmission. Sixty adult Aedes species mosquitoes were airfreighted at -80°Con dry ice to Institute Pasteur in Dakar, Senegal to test for the presence of yellow fever virus by Reverse Transcriptase Polymerase Chain reaction technique.

Sample treatment, processing and testing for yellow fever mosquito vectors

Mosquito species collected as either larvae or pupae were reared to the adult stage and identified using various morphological keys. This meant that larvae and pupae collected in the field were kept at least for 4-6 days to obtain emerging adults. All adult mosquitoes collected from the field were sorted and pooled according to the selected clusters, sex and stored in liquid nitrogen. Adult mosquitoes emerging from the larvae/pupa were sorted accordingly and stored at -80°C until virological tests were completed. For testing of mosquitoes for yellow fever virus, similar species identified were chilled and pooled in maximum 10 mosquitoes per vial and sent to Institute Dakar where they were analysed.

Questionnaire of indoor residual spraying

The human seroprevalence questionnaire contained two questions related to vector control: “Have you slept under a mosquito net the past two weeks?” and “Has your house been sprayed just before the current rainy season?”

Training

Training of field staff was conducted in Ndola in Copperbelt province for a week before the commencement of the main study in North-Western and Western Provinces. The training was facilitated by epidemiologists and medical entomologists, experts from the World health Organisation and Inter-Country Support Team (IST) Harare, Zimbabwe, WHO country office/Zambia, Tropical Diseases Research Centre and Institute Pasteur of Dakar, Senegal facilitated through IST/West Africa.

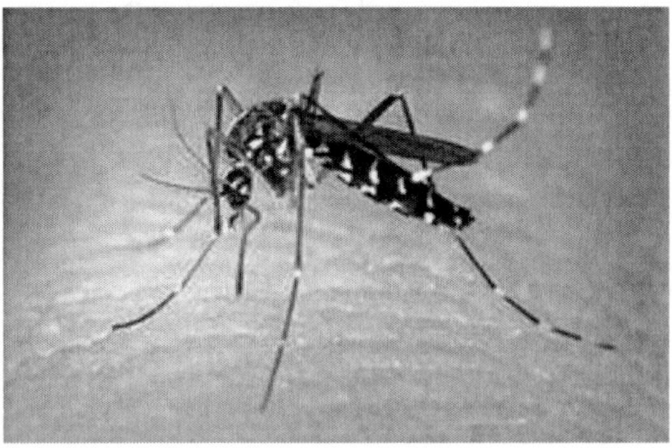

Figure 9. Aedes species.

Entomologic data management and analysis

Vector identification was done using entomological keys (46). Data were stored in Excel software. To assess the entomological epidemic potential of yellow fever disease in Zambia in each selected site we calculated Aedes aegypti (Figure 9) larval density or Breteau index (BI) in domestic environments. The BI (% container positive with larvae/habitation unit) was an indirect measure of vector density which helps to infer an epidemic risk (BI > 5% indicates epidemic risk). We calculated House Index (HI) and Cluster Index (CI). The parameter of container index, which is the percentage of containers where larvae were found, was used to find out the presence of disease-causing mosquitoes. Container index above 10% was considered high and problematic.

Ethical considerations for sampling mosquitoes

Ethical clearance to conduct the survey was granted by the Tropical Diseases Research Centre, Research Ethics Committee. Ethical standards were adhered to throughout this study. All team members involved with the mosquito survey and collection were trained and vaccinated against yellow fever and had prophylactic anti-malarials according to national guidelines. Oral informed consent was obtained from heads of the households in which larval and adult mosquito collection was undertaken. Also, consent was obtained from field collectors participating in entomological assessment. Thus, written informed consent was obtained from all team members and local personnel involved in the mosquito survey and collection.

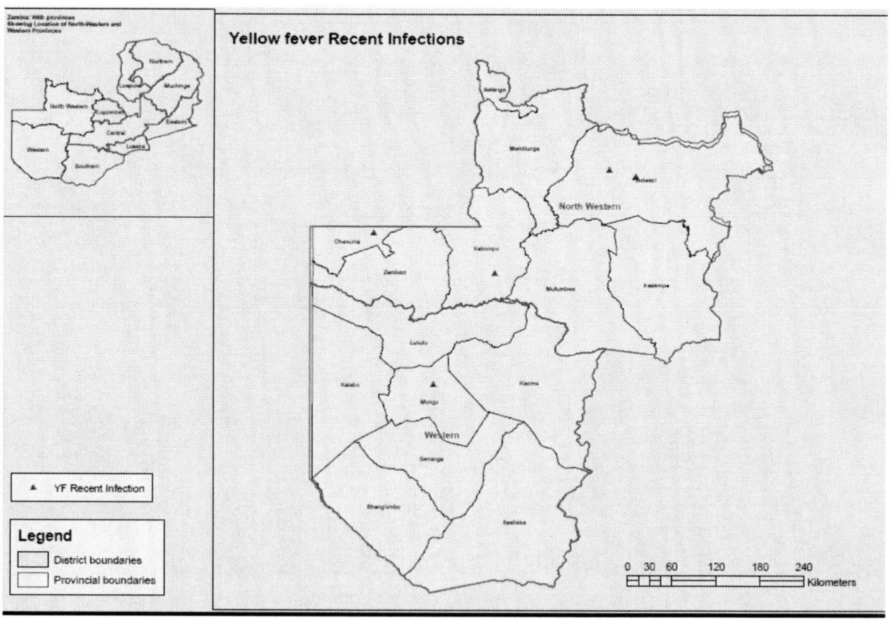

Figure 10. Distribution of recent yellow fever virus infection.

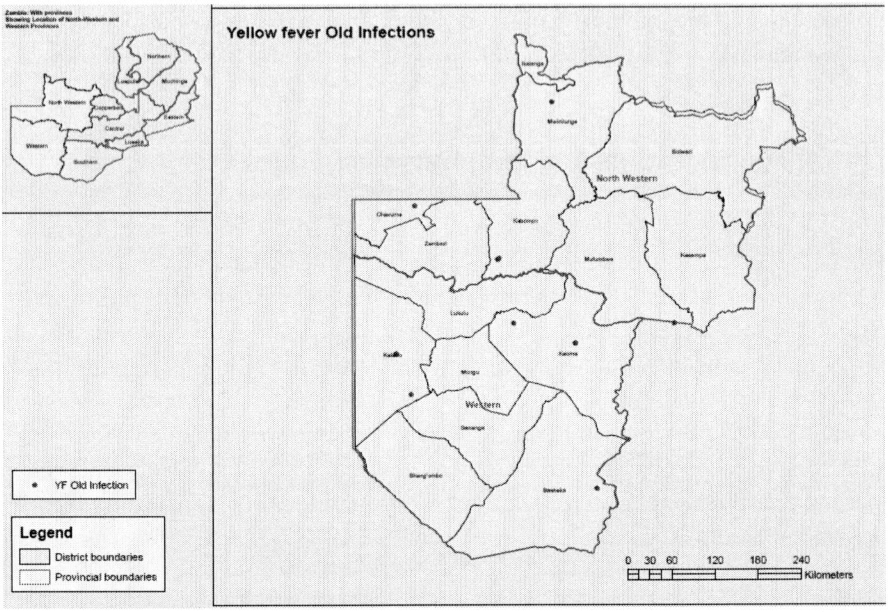

Figure 11. Distribution of old yellow fever virus infection.

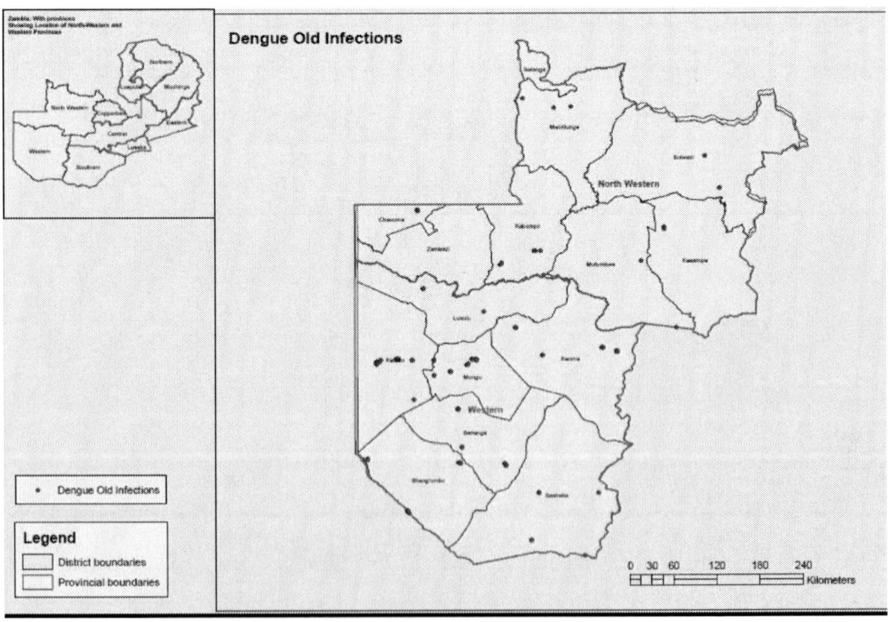

Figure 12. Distribution of old dengue virus infection.

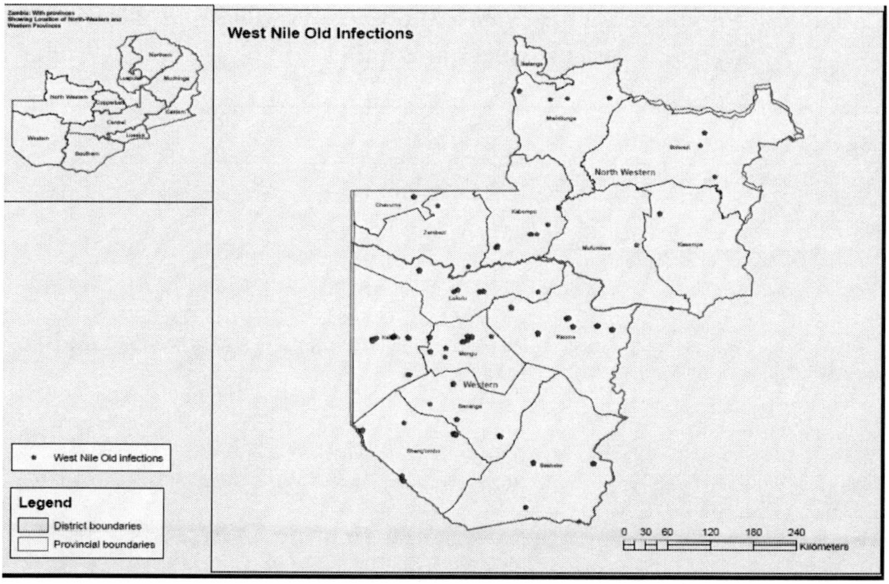

Figure 13. Distribution of old West Nile virus infection.

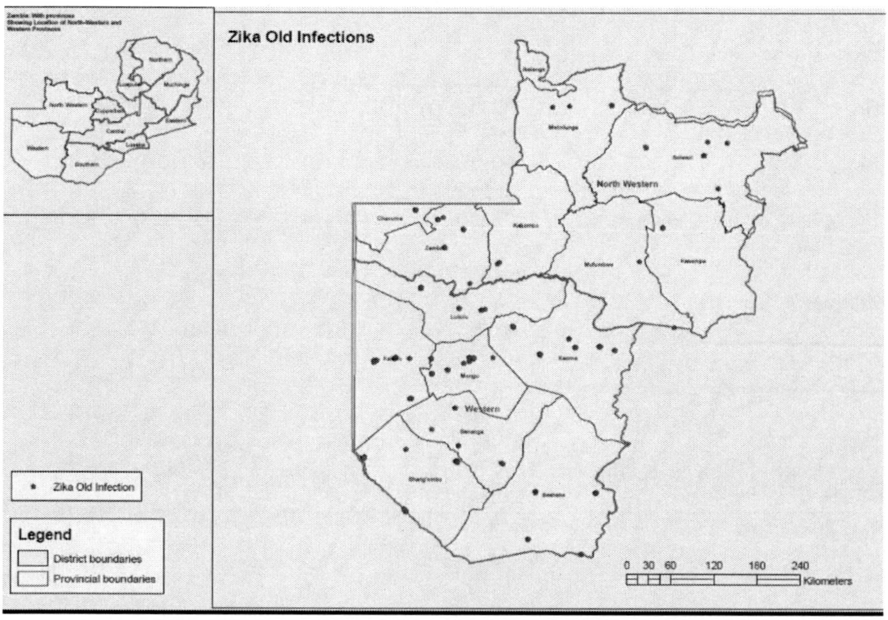

Figure 14. Distribution of old Zika virus infection.

Table 1. Prevalence of arboviruses in North-Western and Western provinces in Zambia

Arboviruses	Total n (%)	Male n (%)	Female n (%)	p value
Yellow fever virus new infections				
Yes	6 (0.2)	4 (0.2)	2 (0.1)	0.427
No	3618 (99.8)	1665 (99.8)	1899 (99.9)	
Yellow fever virus old infections				
Yes	12 (0.3)	8 (0.5)	4 (0.2)	0.246
No	3612 (99.7)	1661 (99.5)	1897 (99.8)	
Prevalence of yellow fever virus infection	**18 (0.5)**	**12 (0.7)**	**6 (0.3)**	**0.101**
Total	3624	1669	1901	
Dengue new infections				
Yes	0 (0)	0 (0)	0(0)	-
No	3624 (100)	1668 (100)	1902 (100)	
Dengue old infections				
Yes	149 (4.1)	69 (4.1)	78 (4.1)	1.000
No	3475 (95.9)	1599 (95.9)	1824 (95.9)	
Prevalence of dengue virus infection	**149 (4.1)**	**69 (4.1)**	**78 (4.1)**	**1.000**
Total	3624	1668	1902	
Total				
West Nile new infections				
Yes	2 (0.1)	2 (0.1)	0 (0)	0.218
No	3623 (99.9)	1667 (99.9)	1902 (100)	
West Nile old infections				
Yes	370 (10.2)	174 (10.4)	195 (10.3)	0.909
No	3255 (89.8)	1495 (89.6)	1707 (89.7)	
Prevalence of West Nile virus infection	**372 (10.3)**	**176 (10.5)**	**195 (10.3)**	**0.817**
Total	3625	1669	1902	
Zika new infections				
Yes	0 (0)	0 (0)	0 (0)	-
No	3625 (100)	1669 (100)	1902 (100)	
Zika old infections				
Yes	217 (6.0)	100 (6.0)	116 (6.1)	0.893
No	3408 (94.0)	1569 (100)	1786 (93.9)	
Prevalence of Zika virus infection	**217 (6.0)**	**100 (6.0)**	**116 (6.1)**	**0.893**
Total	3408 (94.0)	1669	1902	

OUR FINDINGS

The most common arboviruses infections were West Nile (10.3%) and Zika virus infection (6.0%). The prevalence for dengue virus infection was 4.1% and that for yellow fever was 0.5%. No association was observed between sex and arboviruses infection. Both recent and old infections were observed for yellow fever, 0.2% and 0.3%, respectively and West Nile, 0.1% and 10.2%, respectively.

No recent infections were noted for both dengue and Zika virus infection. These results are shown in table 1 and figures 10-14. Altogether, 5 (0.1%) of the participants were positive for all the four arboviruses, 6.3% of the participants were positive for 2 or more arboviruses and 11.5% were positive for any arboviruses (see table 2).

Table 2. Prevalence rates for combinations of arboviruses in North-Western and Western provinces of Zambia

Combinations of arboviruses*	Positive n (%)
0	3206 (88.5)
1	184 (5.1)
2	132 (3.6)
3	96 (2.6)
4	5 (0.1)

* Combinations were for Yellow fever, Dengue, West Nile and Zika viruses.

The study was not powered to conduct correlates for yellow fever. Table 3 shows correlates for dengue, West Nile and Zika arboviruses infection. Consistently, persons aged less than 5 years were about 63% less likely to have any arbovirus infection compared to persons aged 45 years or older. While persons aged 35-44 years were equally likely to have any arbovirus infection as those aged 45 years or older for dengue and Zika, persona aged 35-44 years were 41% more likely to have West Nile virus infection compared to those aged 45 years or older. Education was only significantly related to West Nile virus infection. Participants who attained primary level of education were 32% (AOR= 1.32; 95%CI [1.01-1.72]) more likely to have West Nile virus infection compared to those who attained tertiary level of education. Respondents who were engaged in farming were 20% (AOR=0.80; 95% CI [0.64, 0.99] less likely to have West Nile virus infection compared to respondents who were students.

Table 3. Correlates in multivariate analysis for prevalence of arboviruses in North-Western and Western province of Zambia

	Adjusted odds ratio (95% Confidence interval)		
Factor	Dengue	West Nile	Zika
Age (years)			
<5	0.37 (0.16, 0.86)	0.38 (0.20-0.73)	0.36 (0.18, 0.72)
5-14	0.92 (0.62, 1.38)	0.73 (0.50-1.08)	0.76 (0.54, 1.08)
15-24	0.98 (0.65, 1.47)	1.07 (0.82-1.42)	0.91 (0.64, 1.28)
25-34	1.38 (0.94, 2.03)	1.06 (0.77-1.48)	1.20 0.86, 1.68)
35-44	0.94 (0.59, 1.50)	1.41 (1.01-1.97)	1.27 (0.89, 1.82)
45+	1	1	1
Sex			
Male	-	-	-
Female			
Education			
None	-	0.83 (0.60-1.15)	-
Primary		1.32 (1.01-1.72)	
Secondary		0.98 (0.74-1.30)	
Tertiary		1	
Occupation			
House wife/husband	-	1.13 (0.85-1.51)	-
Farming		0.80 (0.64-0.99)	
Other		1.35 (1.02-1.79)	
Student		1	
Use of an insecticide treated net			
Yes	1.21 (1.01, 1.44)	1.13 (1.00-1.27)	-
No	1	1	
In-door residual spraying			
Yes	-	0.81 (0.69-0.95)	0.81 (0.66, 0.99)
No		1	1
Visited Angola			
Yes	1.73 (1.27, 2.35)	1.40 (1.09, 1.81)	1.42 (1.06, 1.90)
No	1	1	1
Visited DR Congo			
Yes	-	0.28 (0.10, 0.74)	-
No		1	
Roof type			
Grass	2.28 (1.15, 4.53)	2.97 (1.81-4.88)	2.03 (1.24, 3.33)
Iron sheet	0.98 (0.49, 1.99)	0.96 (0.58-1.58)	0.85 (0.51, 1.43)
Asbestos	1	1	1

Participants who used ITNs were more likely to have dengue or West Nile virus infection compared to those who did not use ITNs. Respondents who had in-door residual spraying were 19% less likely to have West Nile or Zika virus infection compared to respondents who did not have in-door residual spraying.

Visiting Angola was significantly associated with increased risk for dengue West Nile and Zika arboviruses infections. Respondents who visited DR Congo were 72% (AOR=0.28; 95% CI [0.10, 0.74]) less likely to have West Nile virus infection compared to those who did not visit DR Congo.

Consistently, participants who stayed in houses that had grass roof were 2-3 times more likely to have any of the arboviruses infection compared to those who lived in houses with asbestos roofs. Participants who lived in houses with iron sheet roof were equally likely to have any arboviruses infection as those who lived in houses with asbestos roof.

A total of 1,401 adult mosquitoes were collected comprising 405 (28.9%) Aedes, 518 (37.0%) Anopheles, 471 (33.6%) Culex and 71 (5.1%) Mansonia. The two main yellow fever vectors found in the study area were Ae.(Stegomyia) aegypti and Ae. (Stegomyia) africanus. Also found in the study area were Aedes (Aedimorphus) mutilus, Ae. (aedimorphus) minutus and Ae. (Finlaya) wellmani.

Discussion

The current study reports a comprehensive distribution of four arboviruses, all of genus Flavivirus, in North-Western and Western provinces. The prevalence rates were 10.3% for West Nile, 6.0% for Zika, 4.1% for dengue and 0.5% for yellow fever. No recent infections were observed for dengue and Zika viruses. In a study conducted in three rural districts of Kenya, Mease et al. (47) reported prevalence rates for West Nile of 9.5%, dengue 14.4% and yellow fever 9.2% in 2004. In the 1966-1968 Kenyan study, the most prevalent arboviruses were West Nile with a prevalence of 23.8%, followed by Zika (17.6%), dengue (17.3%) and lastly yellow fever (14.3%) (30). In another study in rural Cameroon, the prevalence of yellow fever (26.9%) was higher than that for West Nile (6.6%) (48). Dominant arboviruses infections varied in different surveys. Differences in rates may partly be due to different laboratory tests that were conducted and different stages of the epidemic. In the Cameroonian study, the plaque–reduction neutralization test was used. The 2004 Kenyan study used IgG antibodies to test the samples and in the 1966-1968 Kenya study the haemagglutination-inhibition test was used. The Zambian samples were subjected to both IgG and IgM antibody tests and PRNT. Differences in the power of the study may partly explain the different rates that have been observed between studies. Since tests for arboviruses cross react with each other, it is important that confirmatory tests be conducted, and it's none use by some studies may have led to different test results. Given that the study design allowed for computation of point prevalence, the observed rates may be an underestimate for the true prevalence because only those who survived the arboviruses infection were considered in the study.

The finding that about 1 in 20 participants were positive for two or more arboviruses indicates the need to test for more than one arbovirus. This will ensure that patients receive comprehensive management of the infections.

Correlates for arboviruses generally differed between arboviruses, indicating the need to design interventions to control arboviruses infections that are arboviru-specific. However consistently across all the arboviruses, visiting Angola was associated with increased risk for arboviruses. Recently, Angola reported epidemics for Dengue (49). Stoddard et al. (50) and Reiter (51) have argued that human movement is an important factor in the transportation of vectors and pathogens.

The finding that participants aged less than 5 years were less likely to have arboviruses infections compared to older participants cut across all infections suggests that these individuals may have had maternal protection. However, Ministry of Health (52) reported that about a third of children of age 24-59 months had malaria parasites in the 2010 Malaria Indicator Survey, suggesting that children in this age group are susceptible to mosquito bites that may transmit arboviruses. Another finding that cut across all infections was that participants who lived in houses with grass roof type were more likely to have infections compared to those who lived in houses with roofs made of asbestos. It is possible that grass roof type offers favourable house environment for mosquitoes in our study area.

The finding of two main vectors for yellow fever (Ae.(Stegomyia) aegypti and Ae. (Stegomyia) africanus) indicates that there is a possibility of sustaining the virus if it was imported into the study area. Interventions mainly placed for malaria control including insecticide residual spraying and insecticide treated nets are in place but with only about half the population in our study sites using insecticide treated nets (43), the other half of the population or more remain susceptible to arbovirus infections.

We may assume that factors that could have contributed to the risk of arbovirus infection in the population under study include the activities of the vectors, that of the human host and a possible bias in answering the questionnaire on use of ITNs. Aedes aegypti generally bites during the day (53) and therefore the use of ITNs would not be expected to provide a barrier between the humans and the transmitting vector. Considering the outdoor activities participated in during the day such as farming, fishing, and socialising, the population may be at risk of being bitten by the vector.

Worthwhile to note is that subsequent infections with dengue increases the severity of disease and if interventions are not timely put in place, Zambia risks a dengue outbreak. In conclusion, the factors: roof type and visiting Angola in addition to arbovirus-specific correlates should be considered in developing interventions to control arboviruses in North-Western and Western provinces of Zambia.

REFERENCES

[1] Babaniyi OA, Mwaba P, Mulenga D, Monze M, Songolo P, Mazaba-Liwewe ML, et al. Risk assessment for Yellow Fever in Western and North-Western provinces of Zambia. J Global Infect Dis (Ahead of print).

[2] Mazaba-Liwewe ML, Siziya S, Monze M, Mweene-Ndumba I, Masaninga F, Songolo P, et al. First sero-prevalence of dengue fever specific immunoglobulin G antibodies in Western and North-Western provinces of Zambia: a population based cross sectional study. Virol J 2014;11:135.

[3] Lvov DK, Tsyrkin YM, Karas FR, Timopheev EM, Gromashevski VL, Veselovskaya OV, et al. "Sokuluk" Virus, a new group B arbovirus isolated from Vespertilio pipistrellus Schreber, 1775, bat in the Kirghiz S.S.R. Arch Gesamte Virusforschung 1973;41:170-4.

[4] Vainio J, Cutts F. Yellow Fever. WHO Division of Emerging and other Communicable Diseases Surveillance and Control: Geneva: WHO, 1998.

[5] Monath TP. Yellow fever: an update. Lancet Infect Dis 2001;1:11–20.

[6] Julander JG. Experiment therapies for yellow fever. Antiviral Res 2013;97:169-79.

[7] Monath TP. Review of the risks and benefits of yellow fever vaccination including some new analyses. Expert Rev Vaccines 2012;11:427-48.

[8] World Health Organization. Division of Epidemiological Surveillance and Health Situation and Trend Assessment. Global Health Situation and Projections: Estimates. Geneva: World Health Organization, 1992.

[9] World Health Organization. Media centre. Dengue and severe dengue. Fact sheet N°117. Updated March 2014. Accessed 2014 September 12. URL: http://www.who.int/mediacentre/factsheets/fs117/en/)

[10] Simmons CP, Farrar JJ, van Vinh Chau N, Wills B. Dengue. N Engl J Med 2012;366:1423–32.

[11] Whitehorn J, Farrar J. Dengue. Br Med Bull 2010;95:161–73.

[12] World Health Organization, Special Programme for Research and Training in Tropical. Diseases: Dengue: guidelines for diagnosis, treatment, prevention and control. Geneva: World Health Organization, 2009.

[13] Ranjit S, Kissoon N. Dengue hemorrhagic fever and shock syndromes. Pediatr Crit Care Med 2011;12:90–100.

[14] World Health Organization. Dengue and Dengue Hemorrhagic Fever. Fact sheet No117. Revised April 2002. Accessed 2014 September 11: URL: http://shuidao.cn/factSheets/Health_and_Nutrition/whoHealth/whoFS_dengue.pdf

[15] Halstead SB. Dengue vaccine development: a 75% solution? Lancet 2012;380:1535-6.

[16] Sabchareon A, Wallace D, Sirivichayakul C, Limkittikul K, Chanthavanich P, Suvannadabba S, et al. Protective efficacy of the recombinant, live-attenuated, CYD tetravalent dengue vaccine in Thai schoolchildren: a randomised, controlled phase 2b trial. Lancet 2012;380;1559-67.

[17] Bhatt S, Gething PW, Brady OJ, Messina JP, Farlow AW, Moyes CL, et al. The global distribution and burden of dengue. Nature 2013;496:504–7.

[18] Endy TP, Anderson KB, Nisalak A, Yoon IK, Green S, Rothman AL, et al. Determinants of inapparent and symptomatic dengue infection in a prospective study of primary school children in Kamphaeng Phet, Thailand. PLoS Negl Trop Dis 2011;5:e975.

[19] Gubler DJ. Dengue and dengue hemorrhagic fever. Clin Microbiol Rev 1998;11:480–69.

[20] Kakkar M. Dengue fever is massively under-reported in India, hampering our response. Br Med J 2012;345:e8574.

[21] Mostashari F, Bunning ML, Kitsutani PT, Singer DA, Nash D, Cooper MJ, et al. Epidemic West Nile encephalitis, New York, 1999: results of a household-based seroepidemiological survey. Lancet 2001;358:261–4.

[22] Centers for Disease Control and Prevention. West Nile Virus: Symptoms & Treatment. Accessed 2014 September 05. URL: http://www.cdc.gov /westnile/symptoms/.

[23] Centers for Disease Control and Prevention. West Nile Virus: Symptoms & Treatment. Accessed 2014 September 05. URL: http://www.cdc.gov/ westnile/symptoms/.

[24] Rojahn SY. Few Options in the West Nile Fight: The seasonal and unpredictable nature of the infection makes it difficult to test any potential treatment or vaccine. Accessed 2014 September 16. http://www.technologyreview.com/news/428926/few-options-in-the-west-nile-fight/)

[25] Bakonyi T, Nowotny N. West Nile epidemiology: global situation and recent outbreaks in Europe. Workshop on West Nile virus. Berlin, 13th -17th of February, 2012.

[26] European Centre for Disease Prevention and Control. Rapid risk assessment: Zika virus infection outbreak, French Polynesia. 14 February 2014. Stockholm: ECDC, 2014.

[27] Olson JG, Ksiazek TG, Suhandiman, Triwibowo. Zika virus, a cause of fever in Central Java, Indonesia. Trans R Soc Trop Med Hyg 1981;75:389-93.

[28] Heang V, Yasuda CY, Sovann L, Haddow AD, Travassos da Rosa AP, Tesh RB, et al. Zika virus infection, Cambodia, 2010. Emerg Infect Dis 2012;18:349-51.

[29] Duffy MR, Chen TH, Hancock WT, Powers AM, Kool JL, Lanciotti RS, et al. Zika virus outbreak on Yap Island, Federated States of Micronesia. N Engl J Med 2009;360:2536-43.

[30] Geser A, Henderson BE, Christensen S. A multipurpose serological survey in Kenya: 2. Results of arbovirus serological tests. Bull World Health Organ 1970;43:539-52.

[31] Aitken TH, Tesh RB, Beaty BJ, Rosen L. Transovarial transmission of yellow fever virus by mosquitoes (Aedes aegypti). Am J Trop Med Hyg 1979;28:119–21.

[32] Fontenille D, Diallo M, Mondo M, Ndiaye M, Thonnon J. First evidence of natural vertical transmission of yellow fever virus in Aedes aegypti, its epidemic vector. Trans R Soc Trop Med Hyg 1997;91:533–5.

[33] Gratz NG. Critical review of the vector status of Aedes albopictus. Med Vet Entomol 2004;18:215–27.

[34] Masaninga F, Muleba M, Masendu H, Songolo P, Mweene-Ndumba I, Mazaba-Liwewe ML, et al. Distribution of yellow fever vectors in Northwestern and Western Provinces, Zambia. Asian Pac J Trop Biomed 2014; 4(12):(in press).

[35] Kyle JL, Harris E: Global spread and persistence of dengue. Annu Rev Microbiol 2008, 62:71–92.

[36] World Health Organization: Dengue control: the mosquito. Accessed 2014 September 11. URL: http://www.who.int/denguecontrol/mosquito/en/.

[37] Centers for Disease Control and Prevention. Surveillance for West Nile virus disease—United States, 1999–2008. MMWR Surveill Summ 2010;59:1–17.

[38] Reimann C, Hayes E, DiGuiseppi C, Hoffman R, Lehman J, Lindsey N, et al. Epidemiology of neuroinvasive arboviral disease in the United States, 1999–2007. Am J Trop Med Hyg 2008;79:974–9.

[39] Nash D, Mostashari F, Fine A, Miller J, O'Leary D, Murray K, et al. The outbreak of West Nile virus infection in the New York City area in 1999. N Engl J Med 2001;344:1807–14.

[40] Zika Virus Infection. Accessed 2014 September 2014. URL: http://www.

[41] fitfortravel.nhs.uk/advice/disease-prevention-advice/zika-virus-infection.aspx.

[42] Central Statistical Office. 2010 census of population and housing. National analytical report. CSO, 2012.

[43] Aregheore EM. Country pasture/forage resource profiles: Zambia. Accessed 2014 May 19. URL: http://www.fao.org/ag/agp/AGPC/doc/Counprof/zambia/zambia.htm#_Toc131995467.

[44] Central Statistical Office (CSO), Ministry of Health (MOH), Tropical Diseases Research Centre (TDRC), University of Zambia, and Macro International Inc. 2009: Zambia Demographic and Health Survey 2007. Calverton, Maryland, USA: CSO and Macro International Inc, 2011.

[45] Robinson GG. A note on mosquitoes and yellow fever in Northern Rhodesia. East Afr Med J 1950;27:284-8.

[46] World Health Organization. WHO manual for the monitoring of yellow fever virus infection WHO/IVB/04.08. Geneva: World Health Organization, 2004.

[47] Kent RJ. The mosquitoes of Macha, Zambia. Johns Hopkins Malaria Research Institute; Department of Molecular Microbiology and Immunology, Johns Hopkins Bloomberg School of Public Health. Baltimore, MD USA, 2006. Accessed 2014 September 16. URL: http://malaria.jhsph.edu/programs/conferences_workshops/

conference_meetings%20archives/2006%20events/The_Mosquitoes_of_Macha-March06.pdf

[48] Mease LE, Coldren RL, Musila LA, Prosser T, Ogolla F, Ofula VO, et al. Seroprevalence and distribution of arboviral infections among rural Kenyan adults: A cross-sectional study. Virology J 2011;8:371.

[49] Kuniholm MH, Wolfe ND, Huang CY-H, Mpoudi-Ngole E, Tamoufe U, Burke DS, et al. Seroprevalence and distribution of Flaviviridae, Togaviridae, and Bunyaviridae arboviral infections in rural Cameroonian adults. Am J Trop Med Hyg 2006;74:1078–83.

[50] CDC. Ongoing Dengue Epidemic — Angola, June 2013. Morbidity and Mortality Weekly Report (MMWR) 2013;62:504-507. Accessed 2014 September 10. URL: http://www.cdc.gov/mmwr/preview/mmwrhtml/mm6224a6.htm

[51] Stoddard ST, Morrison AC, Vazquez-Prokopec GM, Paz Soldan V, Kochel TJ, Kitron U, et al. The role of human movement in the transmission of vector-borne pathogens. PLoS Negl Trop Dis 2009;3:e481.

[52] Reiter P. Climate change and mosquito-borne disease: knowing the horse before hitching the cart. Rev Sci Tech 2008;27:383-98.

[53] Ministry of Health. Zambia National Malaria Indicator Survey 2010. Lusaka: Ministry of Health, 2010.

[54] Centers for Diseases Control and Prevention: Dengue and the Aedes Aegytpi mosquito. Accessed 2014 September 16. URL: http://www.cdc.gov/dengue/resources/30jan2012/aegyptifactsheet.pdf

In: Arbovirus
Editors: S. Siziya, M. L. Mazaba et al.
ISBN: 978-1-63463-601-8

Chapter 3

PREVALENCE OF YELLOW FEVER

Olusegun Babaniyi, MBBS, MPH, MSc**[*,1]**,
Mazyanga L Mazaba, BSc, MSc**[1]**,
***Freddie Masaninga, BSc, MSc, PhD**[1]**, Peter Mwaba, MBChB, MMed**[2]**, David Mulenga, BSc, MPH**[3]**, Peter Songolo, MBChB, MPH**[1]**, Idah Mweene-Ndumba, BSc, MPH**[1]**, Emmanuel Rudatsikira, MD, MPH, DrPH**[4]**, and Seter Siziya, BA(Ed), MSc, PhD**[3,5]*
[1]World Health Organization, Lusaka, Zambia
[2]Ministry of Home Affairs, Lusaka, Zambia
[3]School of Medicine, Copperbelt University, Ndola, Zambia
[4]School of Health Professions, Andrews University, Michigan, United States of America
[5]University of Lusaka, Lusaka, Zambia

Yellow fever virus infection is a public health problem in Africa. North-Western province of Zambia was reclassified from a no risk to a low risk area for YF in 2010. To ascertain this reclassification, an assessment for the risk of YF was conducted in 2013 in North-Western province. A total of 1,754 persons took part in the survey of which 48.8% were males. Overall, 15.8% of the participants were of age 45 years or older.

* Correspondence: Olusegun A. Babaniyi, MBBS, MPH, MSc, World Health Organization, Lusaka, Zambia. E-mail: agbagba@yahoo.com.

Significantly more males (37.4%) than females (26.0%) had attained secondary or higher levels of education. Nine (0.5%) out of 1,754 participants had YF virus infection. Of the 9 cases, 4 were old infection and 5 were new. There were 6 Male and 3 female cases. The age range of the cases was 37-81 years. None of the cases had jaundice or bled but 3 had fever. Three cases had travelled to Congo DR and 1 case had travelled to Angola. Use of mosquito net was reported by 4 cases and another 4 cases reported that their houses were sprayed with IRS. The prevalence of YF virus infection among participants of ages 45 years or older (2.9%) was significantly ($p<0.001$) higher than that for participants aged less than 45 year (0.1%). North-Western province was experiencing an epidemic for YF virus infection. With a low prevalence, the area qualifies to be classified as a low risk for YF. Efforts to curb the epidemic are urgently needed. Yellow fever surveillance and the capacity of laboratories to diagnose YF should be strengthened.

INTRODUCTION

Yellow fever virus infection is a public health problem in Africa. Epidemics of YF have spread from West Africa (1,2) where 13 of 14 west African countries reported YFV infection from 2000 to 2006 (3,4,5) to North Africa (6), East Africa (7), Central Africa and Southern Africa (8).

Yellow fever affects about 200000 people annually in the tropics of Africa and South America (9). Symptoms for YF virus infection includes: fever, chills, severe headache, back pain, general body aches, nausea, vomiting, fatigue and weakness to severe liver disease with bleeding. About 15% of cases progress to a more severe form of the disease that is characterized by high fever, jaundice, bleeding, and eventually shock and failure of multiple organs (10). There is no treatment for yellow fever and only symptoms can be alleviated. YF virus infection can be prevented by using insect repellent, wearing protective clothing, and getting vaccinated.

Although by 2005, Yellow fever was endemic in Congo DR, the area of Congo DR bordering North-Western was classified as a low risk area for YF (11). North-Western province of Zambia was reclassified by WHO from a no risk area to a low risk area for YF in 2010 (8). To ascertain this reclassification, an assessment for the risk of YF was conducted in 2013 in North-Western province.

OUR STUDY

The study was conducted in North-Western province of Zambia. North-Western province borders with Angola on the western side and Democratic Republic of Congo (DRC) on the northern side with 6 districts divided into 1,178 Standard Enumeration Areas (SEAs). The 2010 census reveals a population of 706,462 with population density of 5.6 (12). The main economic activity was pineapple growing, with fast growing mining activities. Zambia Demographic Health Survey, 2007 reports 46.9 and 53.2% of the population sleeping under a net in the past night in Western and North Western Provinces respectively (13).

This assessment was carried out among individuals aged nine months or older. The sample size calculation was based on the assumption that the sero-prevalence was 7% based on the study conducted by Robinson (14).

In estimating the sample size for persons aged 5 years or older, the following parameters were considered: a prevalence of 7%, desired precision or confidence interval (d) of $\pm$3%, and a design effect (DE) of 2 and an 80% response rate. Considering sex, we aimed to recruit 700 male and 700 female participants in each province. Assuming an average of 4 persons aged 5 years or older in each household, a total of 12 households in each of the 30 cluster were to be recruited in the survey. The total number of persons that would be recruited was 1806.

The sero-prevalence of children was about half that for older children, and in estimating the sample size for persons aged below 5 years, the following parameters were considered: a prevalence of 3.5%, desired precision or confidence interval (d) of $\pm$3.4%, and a design effect (DE) of 2 and an 80% response rate. The computed sample size was 282. Therefore, 406 children would be recruited for the survey.

The sample was drawn using a two-stage cluster sampling technique using probability proportional to size. A list of the standard enumeration areas (SEAs) in each province constituted the sampling frame.

Data were entered in an Epi-Info data entry screen that had consistency and range checks embedded in it. Further editing was conducted by running frequencies during the analysis stage. Epi data files were exported to SPSS for data analysis. The chi-square test was used to determine associations between qualitative factors. The cut off point for statistical significance was set at the 5% level.

Ethical clearance was sought from the Tropical Diseases Research Centre Research Ethics Committee, and ethical standards were adhered to throughout this study. Informed consent was sought from study participants. Guardians provided assent for the participation of the persons under the consenting age. They were asked to read or have read to them, understand and sign/thumbprint an informed consent form. Responsible adults in the household were identified to give proxy consent on behalf of minors.

OUR FINDINGS

A total of 1,754 persons took part in the survey of which 48.8% were males. Overall, 15.8% of the participants were of age 45 years or older. Significantly more males (37.4%) than females (26.0%) had attained secondary or higher levels of education. These results are shown in table 1.

Table 1. Sample description for the participants in yellow fever risk assessment, 2013

Factor	Total n (%)	Male n (%)	Female n (%)	p value
Age (years)				
<45	1476 (84.2)	703 (82.4)	2769 (85.7)	0.067
45+	278 (15.8)	150 (17.6)	128 (14.3)	
Sex				
Male	854 (48.8)	-	-	
Female	897 (51.2)			
Education				
None or primary	1182 (68.4)	525 (62.6)	654 (74.0)	<0.001
Secondary or higher	545 (31.6)	314 (37.4)	230 (26.0)	
Yellow fever				
Yes	9 (0.5)	6 (0.7)	3 (0.3)	0.459
No	1745 (99.5)	848 (99.3)	893 (99.7)	

Nine (0.5%) out of 1754 participants had YF virus infection. Of the 9 cases, 4 were old infection and 5 were new. There were 6 Male and 3 female cases. The age range of the cases was 37-81 years. None of the cases had jaundice or bled but 3 had fever.

Three of the cases had no formal education, 4 attained primary level of education and 2 attained secondary level of education. Three cases lived in houses that had roofs made of grass, 5 had roofs made of iron sheets and 1 lived in a house that had a roof made of asbestos. Walls for houses for the cases were made of mud (2), cement plastered (10 and unburnt bricks (6).

Three cases had travelled to Congo DR and 1 case had travelled to Angola. Use of mosquito net was reported by 4 cases and another 4 cases reported that their houses were sprayed with IRS.

None of the factors considered in the analysis was significantly associated with YF virus infection except age. The prevalence of YF virus infection among participants of ages 45 years or older (2.9) was significantly ($p<0.001$) higher than that for participants aged less than 45 year (0.1%).

DISCUSSION

Yellow fever virus was circulating in North-Western province with a prevalence of 0.5%. Both new and old cases were identified in the study area. All the cases of Yellow fever were adults and none of the cases had been vaccinated against YF virus. This survey was conducted 50 years after the last survey of YF virus risk assessment was conducted.

The prevalence of the infection in the current study is less than the 7% that was reported by Robinson (14). The difference in the prevalence could partly be due to differences in the stages of the epidemic at the time of the survey. It might be that North-Western province was in the early stage of the epidemic, while 50 years ago when that study was conducted the area was at an advanced stage of the epidemic. Another possibility for the difference could be that Western province that is not part of the current study could have had a higher proportion of the 7% prevalence.

All the cases of YF in the current study were adults. This finding contradicts the observation that children are more affected than adults because adults could have acquired immunity in a Yellow fever endemic area (15). However, the finding in the current study that adults were more affected is in agreement with the finding by Geser et al. (16) which suggests that stable rates of transmission in the population.

In conclusion, North-Western province was experiencing an epidemic for YF virus infection. With a low prevalence, the area qualifies to be classified as a low risk for YF. Efforts to curb the epidemic are urgently needed. Yellow fever surveillance and the capacity of laboratories to diagnose YF should be strengthened.

Acknowledgments

We are grateful to the interviewers for their dedicated work to successfully complete the survey. The survey could not have been successful without the cooperation of the participants and the virology laboratory staff both in Lusaka, Zambia and Dakar, Senegal for in testing samples. The survey was funded by the Ministry of Health [Zambia] and the World Health Organization.

References

[1] Nasidi A, Monath TP, DeCock K, Tomori O, Cordellier R, Olaleye OD, et al. Urban yellow fever epidemic in western Nigeria, 1987. Trans R Soc Trop Med Hyg 1989;83:401–6.

[2] Robertson SE, Hull BP, Tomori O, Bele O, LeDuc JW, Esteyes K. Yellow fever: a decade of reemergence. JAMA 1996; 276:1157-62.

[3] World Health Organization. Yellow fever vaccine: WHO position paper. Wkly Epidemiol Rec 2003;78:349-59.

[4] Nathan N, Barry M, Van Herp M, Zeller H. Shortage of vaccines during a yellow fever outbreak in Guinea. Lancet 2001;358:2129-30.

[5] Anonymous. The yellow fever situation in Africa and South America in 2004. Wkly Epidemiol Rec 2005;80:249-56.

[6] Gould LH, Osman MS, Farnon EC, Griffith KS, Godsey MS, Karch S, et al. An outbreak of yellow fever with concurrent chikungunya virus transmission in South Kordofan, Sudan, 2005. Trans R Soc Trop Med Hyg 2008;102:1247-54.

[7] Sanders EJ, Marfin AA, Tukei PM, Kuria G, Ademba G, Agata NN, et al. First recorded outbreak of yellow fever in Kenya, 1992-1993. I. Epidemiologic investigations. Am J Trop Med Hyg 1998;59:644-9.

[8] Jentes ES, Poumerol G, Gershman MD, Hill DR, Lemarchand J, Lewis RF, et al. The revised global yellow fever risk map and recommendations for vaccination, 2010: consensus of the Informal WHO Working Group on Geographic Risk for Yellow Fever. Lancet Infect Dis 2011;11:622-32.

[9] Vainio J, Cutts F. Yellow fever. In: World Health Organization. Expanded Programme on Immunization. Global Programme for Vaccines and Immunization: Expanded Programme on Immunization. Geneva: Global Programme for Vaccines and Immunization, Expanded Programme on Immunization, World Health Organization, 1998.

[10] Centers for Disease Control and Prevention. Symptoms and treatment. Accessed 2014 August 28. URL:http://www.cdc.gov/yellowfever/symptoms/index.html

[11] Barnett ED. Yellow fever: epidemiology and prevention. Clin Infect Dis 2007;44:850-6

[12] Central Statistical Office. 2010 census of population and housing. National analytical report. Lusaka, Zambia: CSO, 2012.

[13] Central Statistical Office (CSO), Ministry of Health (MOH), Tropical Diseases Research Centre (TDRC), University of Zambia, and Macro International Inc. 2009. Zambia Demographic and Health Survey 2007. Calverton, Maryland, USA: CSO and Macro International Inc.

[14] Robinson GG. A note on mosquitoes and yellow fever in Northern Rhodesia. East Afr Med J 1950;27:284-8.

[15] Monath TP, Craven RB, Adjukiewicz A, et al. Yellow fever in the Gambia, 1978-1979: epidemiologic aspects with observations on the occurrence of Orungo virus infection. Am J Trop Med Hyg 1980;29:912-28.

[16] Geser A, Henderson BE, Christensen S. A multipurpose serological survey in Kenya: 2. Results of arbovirus serological tests. Bull World Health Organ 1970;43:539-52.

In: Arbovirus ISBN: 978-1-63463-601-8
Editors: S. Siziya, M. L. Mazaba et al.

Chapter 4

DENGUE IGG SEROPREVALENCE

***Mazyanga L Mazaba, BSc, MSc**[*1,2]**, Olusegun Babaniyi, MBBS, MPH, MSc**[1]**, Mwaka Monze, MBChB, PhD**[2]**, Idah Mweene-Ndumba, BSc, MPH**[1,2]**, Freddie Masaninga, BSc, MSc, PhD**[1]**, Peter Songolo, MBChB, MPH**[1]**, Muzala Kanyanga, MBChB, MPH**[3]**, and Seter Siziya, BA(Ed), MSc, PhD**[4,5]*

[1]World Health Organization Country Office, Lusaka
[2]University Teaching Hospital, Lusaka, Zambia. mazmazli@yahoo.com.
[3]Ministry of Health, Lusaka, Zambia
[4]School of Medicine, Copperbelt University, Ndola, Zambia
[5]University of Lusaka, Lusaka, Zambia

The factors associated with Dengue fever may not be well understood but documentation cites an association with demographic and societal changes over the past 50 years. Information on dengue virus infection in North-Western province is lacking. The objective of the study was to determine the prevalence and correlates for dengue virus infection in the province. Secondary data obtained in a yellow fever risk assessment was used in the study. Logistic regression analysis was used to determine magnitudes of associations. A total of 1,755 participants had both

---

[*] Correspondence: Mazyanga L Mazaba, EPI Unit, World Health Organization, Lusaka, Zambia and Virology Unit, University Teaching Hospital, Lusaka, Zambia. E-mail: mazmazli@yahoo.com.

laboratory results and filled in the questionnaires. The results indicated that 1.0% of participants had previous dengue infection with no sex difference (p=0.729). Visiting Angola was significantly associated with previous dengue infection (OR= 2.73; 95% CI [1.55, 4.83]). This study provides evidence of dengue virus circulation and its association with travel to Angola. There is need for active surveillance and adequate diagnostic systems.

INTRODUCTION

Dengue fever caused by dengue virus of genus *Flavivirus* and family *Flaviviridae* is a leading cause of morbidity and mortality in the tropics and subtropics posing a risk to one third of the world's population living in these areas (1, 2). The virus is transmitted to humans through the bite of a mosquito, primarily Aedes Aegypti and Aedes albopictus (2). Until the middle of the 20th century, dengue was a relatively minor, geographically restricted disease (3-4). Pandemic Dengue begun in Southeast Asia in the mid 1940's after the second World War, has intensified in the last 15 years, (5) and has become endemic in more than 100 countries in Africa, the Americas, the Eastern Mediterranean, South-east Asia and the Western Pacific with the American, South-east Asia and the Western Pacific regions affected most seriously (6-8). Based on data submitted by WHO member states mostly affected by dengue indicates cases exceeding 1.2 million in 2008 and 2.3 million in 2010 (9). In Africa, documentation indicates dengue epidemics occurring as far back as 1927 (10) and increasing activity since 1980 (11). Angola and Kenya continued to experience dengue outbreaks in 2013 (12).

The factors associated with Dengue fever may not be well understood but documentation cites an association with demographic and societal changes over the past 50 years (13, 14). Factors including sex, age, urbanization and mobility of people have been associated with increased dengue fever.

The difference in incidence of dengue fever in relation to sex is attributed exposure to the vector (mosquito) (15). Most studies indicate risk of dengue fever increasing with age, urbanization and travel (9, 16-20). Older children and adults are more disposed to dengue fever (6). WHO documents that the increased mobility of people has contributed to the increase in the number of epidemics and circulating viruses (9).

Persons with chronic diseases including diabetes and asthma are likely to encounter complicated disease which is life threatening (21). Once infected with dengue, IgG antibodies and detectable after 10 to 14 days of onset and one acquires lifetime immunity to the specific serotype. Infection with another serotype also increases chances of severity (22). This paper describes the association, if any, of factors including age, sex, education and travel with dengue fever in North-Western province of Zambia.

OUR STUDY

North-Western province borders with Angola on the western side and Democratic Republic of Congo (DRC) (see figure 1) on the northern side with 6 districts divided into 1,178 Standard Enumeration Areas (SEAs). The 2010 census reveals a population of 706,462 with population density of 5.6. The main economic activity was pineapple growing, with fast growing mining activities in one of the districts, Solwezi (23). Central Statistical Office (CSO) (24) reported in 2007 that 53.2% of the population slept under a net in the past night in North-Western province (24).

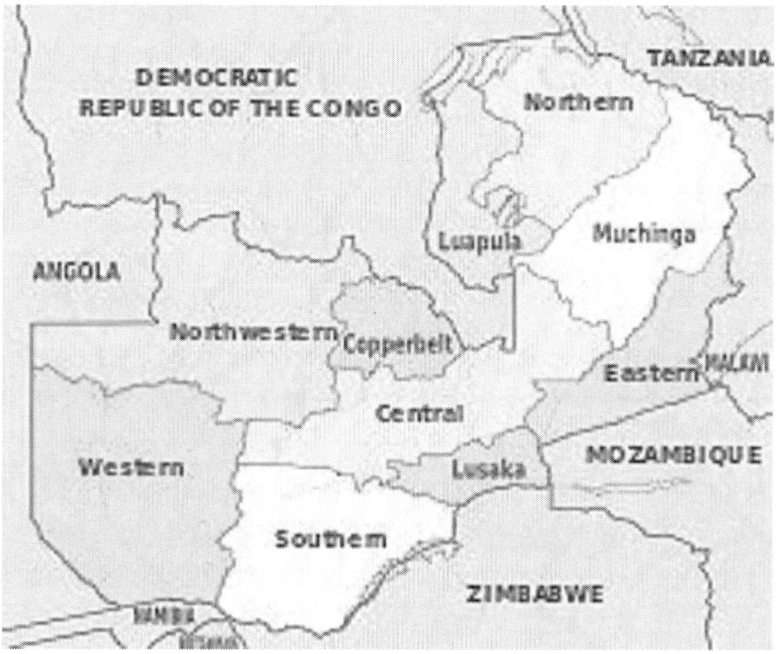

Figure 1. Map of Zambia showing provinces and bordering countries.

Study population, Sample size, inclusion/exclusion criteria and sampling

This assessment was carried out among individuals aged nine months or older. The sample size calculation was based on the assumption that the sero-prevalence was 7% based on the study on Yellow fever conducted by Robinson, 1950 (25). For persons aged 5 years or older the following parameters were considered in estimating the sample size, a prevalence of 7%, desired precision or confidence interval (d) of $\pm$3%, and a design effect (DE) of 2 and an 80% response rate. The study aimed to recruit 700 male and 700 female participants in each province. A total of 12 households in each of the 30 clusters, assuming an average of 4 persons aged 5 years or older in each household, were to be recruited in the survey. The total number of persons that would be recruited from each province was 1,806, totalling 3,612 from both provinces.

The sero-prevalence of children below five years was about half that for older children, and in estimating the sample size for persons aged below 5 years, the following parameters were considered: a prevalence of 3.5%, desired precision or confidence interval (d) of $\pm$3.4%, and a design effect (DE) of 2 and an 80% response rate. The computed sample size was 282. A total of 406 children would be recruited in each province for the survey.

Any individual aged 9 months or older and who was a member of a sampled household and resident in the study site for at least seven days. Individuals who received YF vaccination in the last ten years would be eligible to participate in the survey. Exclusion criteria left out any person, who was either less than 9 months of age, or any person regardless of age, who resided in the study site for a period of less than seven days prior to the survey. Children under the age of nine months raises the risk of false positive results as children under this age may still carry maternal antibodies from immunized or exposed mothers.

A two-stage cluster sampling technique using probability proportional to size was used to draw the sample. A list of the standard enumeration areas (SEAs) in each province constituted the sampling frame. The sampling was designed to achieve fairly good estimates at the provincial level of analysis, and not representing the subdivisions of the province.

Study variables

Dependent variable

A case with evidence of Dengue infection exposure was defined as any individual aged 9 months or older whose blood sample was confirmed to have Dengue virus exposure through the detection of Dengue virus-specific IgG and IgM antibodies.

Independent variables

The independent variables included age, sex, occupation, history of travel to Angola and/or DRC, and use of mosquito preventive measures.

Laboratory procedure

About 3 to 5 millilitres of blood was collected by venepuncture into an EDTA vacutainer tube and transported on cold chain to the local laboratories for serum separation and storage. Samples were subjected to primary testing (YFV specific IgG and IgM) at the University of Teaching Hospital in Zambia virology unit and Institute Pasteur, Dakar. All presumptive YFV-specific IgG and IgM samples were subjected to IgG and IgM antibodies against other flaviviruses known to cause haemorrhagic fever-like disease including dengue.

Data management and analysis

Data were entered in an Epi-Info data entry screen that had consistency and range checks embedded in it. Further editing was conducted by running frequencies during the analysis stage. Epi data files were exported to SPSS for data analysis. The data was summarized to describe the occurrence of dengue virus exposed individuals in absolute numbers and percentage by place (residence, travel or work) and person (age, sex, occupation). Further analysis was conducted to determine independent factors associated with yellow fever sero-positivity. Odds ratios were used to estimate the magnitude of associations.

Ethical considerations

Ethical clearance was sought from the Tropical Diseases Research Centre Research Ethics Committee, and ethical standards were adhered to throughout this study. Informed consent was sought from study participants. Guardians provided assent for the participation of the persons under the consenting age. They were asked to read or have read to them, understand and sign/thumbprint an informed consent form. Responsible adults in the household were identified to give proxy consent on behalf of minors.

Table 1. Sample description for North-Western provinces for dengue virus infection

Factor	Total n (%)	Male n (%)	Female n (%)
Age (years)	[$x^2 = 7.79$, $p = 0.168$]		
<15	533 (30.4)	267 (31.3)	265 (29.5)
15-24	348 (19.8)	164 (19.2)	182 (20.3)
25-34	348 (19.8)	151 (17.7)	197 (22.0)
35-44	247 (14.1)	121 (14.2)	125 (13.9)
45+	278 (15.8)	150 (17.6)	128 (14.3)
Sex			
Male	854 (48.8)	-	-
Female	897 (51.2)	-	-
Education	[$x^2 = 26.22$, $p < 0.001$]		
None	370 (21.4)	160 (19.1)	209 (23.6)
Primary	812 (47.0)	365 (43.5)	445 (50.3)
Secondary or higher	545 (31.6)	314 (37.4)	230 (26.0)
Dengue virus Infection	[$x^2 = 0.12$, $p = 0.729$]		
Yes	18 (1.0)	10 (1.2)	8 (0.9)
No	1737 (99.0)	844 (99.8)	889 (99.1)

OUR FINDINGS

A total of 1755 participants had both laboratory results and filled in the questionnaires. The sample comprised 48.8% females. Overall, 30.4% of the participants were aged less than 15 years. Male participants tended to have attained higher education levels than females (p<0.001). The results indicated 1.0% previous dengue infection amongst the participants in North-Western province. No significant association was observed between sex and dengue infection (p=0.729). These results are shown in table 1. Of the factors considered in bivariate analyses (Table 2), only visit to Angola was significantly associated with previous dengue infection (OR= 2.73; 95% CI [1.55, 4.83]).

DISCUSSION

This study reveals that 1.0% of the study population in North-western had dengue IgG antibodies, indicating having past exposure to dengue infection. A retrospective study on German expatriates who worked in endemic countries for an average of 10 years revealed 4.3% dengue IgG response (26). A prospective study on 104 long term Israel travellers to dengue endemic areas indicated a dengue seroprevalence of 6.7% (27).

Table 2. Factors associated with Dengue virus infection in logistic regression analysis for Western province

Factor	OR (95% CI)
Age (years)	
<15	0.61 (0.21, 1.71)
15-24	0.31 (0.06, 1.55)
25-34	1.24 (0.48, 3.19)
35-44	2.21 (0.91, 5.33)
45+	1
Sex	
Male	1.15 (0.72, 1.83)
Female	1
Education	
None	0.81 (0.35, 1.87)
Primary	1.11.(0.59, 2.11)
Secondary or higher	1
Use of mosquito net	
Yes	1.41 (0.84, 2.37)
No	1
Insecticide Residual Spraying	
Yes	1.30 (0.8, 2.09)
No	1
Visited Angola	
Yes	2.73 (1.55, 4.83)
No	1

Of the factors investigated including age, sex, education and travel to Angola and or Democratic Republic of Congo (DRC), only travel to Angola was positively associated with exposure to dengue infection. Various studies have indicated travel as a significant factor in dengue infection.

Wilder-Smith and Gubler (28) described travel as having the most impact for the spread of dengue from one region to another. They documented that epidemics of dengue, its seasonality and oscillations over time are reflected in the epidemiology of dengue in travellers (29). In a study on travellers returning from endemic countries, dengue infection was associated with 7-45% of cases of fever (30).

Among the countries with evidence of on-going dengue outbreaks including Angola, Democratic Republic of Congo, Mozambique, Tanzania and Seychelles, all except Seychelles neighbour Zambia. The North-Western province of Zambia shares the border with Angola and DRC (Figure 1). This boundary, like most in Africa tends to divide villages, with inhabitants of the same family living on either side of the border. Small scale trade, and search for medical facilities necessitates frequent travels across the border and this could be a contributing factor to spread of disease including dengue.

It is safe to assume the continued circulation of dengue in Angola is associated with sero-prevalence in North-Western province of Zambia, considering its proximity to Angola and a significant association of Dengue infection with travel to Angola. Mazaba-Liwewe et al. indicated presence of dengue IgG antibodies in Western province of Zambia, which borders North-Western province on the southern side and also borders with Angola (31). There may also be transmission of dengue virus between the two provinces of Zambia.

Limitations in this study lie in the fact that plaque reduction neutralization tests (PRNTs) to increase the specificity of ELISA testing and reduce potential cross reactivity were not performed. Although the IgG capture-ELISA test used is a suitable tool to detecting Dengue IgG antibodies in large epidemiologic surveys (32), caution must be taken considering that cross-reactivity may occur with other Flavivirus antibodies (33).

CONCLUSION

This study provides evidence of dengue virus circulation in North-Western provinces of Zambia. It also elaborates on an important factor of association with travel to Angola which is a dengue endemic area. Dengue is a disease of public health importance especially that subsequent infection with other serotypes may lead to more severe cases and fatalities. There is need for active surveillance and adequate diagnostic systems considering how porous the borders with the endemic countries are.

ACKNOWLEDGMENTS

We acknowledge the laboratory support received from Virology laboratory staff (Cynthia Mubanga-Phiri, Julia Chibumbya and Hope Nkamba), University Teaching Hospital, Lusaka, Zambia and Institute de Pasteur, Dakar, Senegal. We are grateful to the interviewers for their dedicated work to successfully complete the survey. The survey could not have been successful without the cooperation of the participants. The survey was funded by the Ministry of Health [Zambia] and the World Health Organization for field activities.

All authors have approved the submission and declare that they have no competing interests.

REFERENCES

[1] US Centers for Disease Control (CDC). Accessed February 2014. URL: http://www.cdc.gov/dengue/.

[2] US Centers for Disease Control (CDC). Accessed February 2014. URL: http://www.nc.cdc.gov/travel/yellowbook/2014/chapter-3-infectious-diseases-related-to-travel/dengue.

[3] US Centers for Disease Control (CDC). Accessed February 2014. URL:http://www.cdc.gov/Dengue/epidemiology/index.html.

[4] Bhatt S, Gething PW, Brady OJ, Messina JP, Farlow AW, Moyes CL, et al. The global distribution and burden of dengue. Nature 2013;496(7446):504-7.

[5] Gubler DJ, Clark GG. Dengue/Dengue hemorrhagic fever: The emergence of a global health problem. Emerg Infect Dis 1995;2: 55-7.

[6] Gubler DJ. Dengue and Dengue hemorrhagic fever. Clin Microbiol Rev 1998;11(3):480.

[7] Hayes EB, Gubler DJ. Dengue and dengue hemorrhagic fever. Pediatr Infect Dis J 1992;11:311–7.

[8] Ranjit S, Kissoon N. Dengue hemorrhagic fever and shock syndromes. Pediatr Crit Care Med 2011;12(1):90–100.

[9] World Health Organization. Dengue and severe dengue fact sheet. Accessed 4 February 2014. URL:http://www.who.int/mediacentre/factsheets/fs117/en/index.html

[10] Sang RC. Dengue in Africa. Accessed 28 February, 2014.URL: http://www. tropika.net/svc/review/061001-Dengue_in_Africa. Tropika.net 2007.

[11] Gubler DJ. Dengue. In: Monath TPM, ed. Epidemiology of arthropodborne viral disease. Boca Raton, FL: CRC Press, 1988:223-60.

[12] Schwartz E, Meltzer E, Mendelson M, Tooke A, Steiner F, Gautret P, et al. Detection on four continents of dengue fever cases related to an ongoing outbreak in Luanda, Angola, March to May 2013. Euro Surveill 2013;18(21): pii-20488.

[13] Gubler DJ. Dengue and dengue hemorrhagic fever in the Americas. P R Health Sci J 1987;6:107–11.

[14] Gubler DJ. Dengue and dengue hemorrhagic fever. Semin Pediatr Infect Dis 1997;8:1.

[15] Anker M, Amina Y. Male-female differences in the number of reported incident dengue fever cases in six Asian countries. Western Pac Surveill Response J 2011;2(2):17-23.

[16] Egger ER, Coleman PG. Age and clinical dengue illness. Emerg Infect Dis 2007;13(6):924-5.

[17] Hayes EB, Gubler DJ. Dengue and dengue hemorrhagic fever. Pediatr Infect Dis J 1992;11:311–7.

[18] Teixera MG, Costa Mda C, Barreto ML. Dengue: twenty-five years since reemergence in Brazil. Cad Saude Publica 2009;25(suppl 1):S7-18.

[19] Cavalcanti LP, Vilar D, Santos RS, Teixeira MG. Change in age pattern of persons with Dengue, northeastern Brazil [letter]. Emerg Infect Dis 2011;7(1):132-4.

[20] Blackburn NK, Rawat R. Dengue fever imported from India: A report of 3 cases SAMJ 1987;71:386-7.

[21] Guzman MG, Halstead SB, Artsob H, Buchy P, Farrar J, Gubler DJ, et al. Dengue: a continuing global threat. Nature Rev Microbiol 2010;8(12Suppl):S7–S16.doi:10.1038/nrmicro246.

[22] Gubler DJ. Dengue and dengue haemorrhagic fever. Clin Microbiol Rev 1998;11(3):480-96.

[23] Civil Society for Poverty Reduction. 2013 report. Accessed February 2014. URL: http://www.csprzambia.org/.

[24] Central Statistical Office (CSO), Ministry of Health (MOH), Tropical Diseases Research Centre (TDRC), University of Zambia, and Macro International Inc. Zambia Demographic and Health Survey 2007. Calverton, MD: CSO, Macro International, 2009.

[25] Robinson GG. A note on mosquitoes and yellow fever in Northern Rhodesia. East Afr Med J 1950;27(7):284-8.

[26] Potasman I, Srugo I, Schwartz E. Dengue seroconversion among Israeli travelers to tropical countries. Emerg Infect Dis 1999;5(6):824-7.

[27] Groen J, Koraka P, Velzing J, Corprac, Osterhaus AD. Evaluation of six immunoassays for detection of dengue virus specific immunoglobulin M and G antibodies. Clin Diagn Lab Immunol 2000;7(6):867-71.

[28] Wilder-Smith A, Gubler DJ. Geographic expansion of dengue: the impact of international travel. Med Clin North Am 2008;92(6):1377-90.

[29] Cobelens FG, Groen J, Osterhaus AD, Leentvaar-Kuipers A, Wertheim-van Dillen PM, Kager PA. Incidence and risk factors of probable dengue virus infection among Dutch travellers to Asia. Trop Med Int Health 2002;7(4):331-8.

[30] Jänisch T, Preiser W, Berger A, Niedrig M, Mikulicz U, Thoma B, et al. Emerging viral pathogens in long-term expatriates (II): Dengue virus. Trop Med Int Health 1997;2(10):934-40.

[31] Mazaba-Liwewe ML, Siziya S, Monze M, Mweene-Ndumba I, Masaninga F, Songolo P, et al. First sero-prevalence of dengue fever specific immunoglobulin G antibodies in Western and North-Western provinces of Zambia: a population based cross sectional study. Virol J 2014;11:135.

[32] Groen J, Koraka P, Velzing J, Copra C, Osterhaus AD. Evaluation of six immunoassays for detection of dengue virus-specific immunoglobulin M and G antibodies. Clin Diagn Lab Immunol 2000;7: 867-71.

[33] Ha DQ, Huong VTQ, Loan HTK, Thang DQ, Duebel V. Seroprevalence of dengue antibodies, annual incidence and risk factors among children in southern Vietnam. Trop Med Int Health 2005;10:379-86.

In: Arbovirus
Editors: S. Siziya, M. L. Mazaba et al.
ISBN: 978-1-63463-601-8

Chapter 5

ZIKA VIRUS INFECTION SPECIFIC IGG IN NORTH-WESTERN PROVINCE OF ZAMBIA

Olusegun Babaniyi, MBBS, MPH, MSc[1],
Peter Songolo, MBChB, MPH*[1],
Mazyanga L Mazaba, BSc, MSc[1],
Idah Mweene-Ndumba, BSc, MPH[1],
Freddie Masaninga, BSc, MSc, PhD[1],
Emmanuel Rudatsikira, MD, MPH, DrPH[2],
and Seter Siziya, BA-Ed, MSc, PhD[3,4]
[1]World Health Organization, Lusaka, Zambia
[2]School of Health Professionals, Andrews University, Michigan, United States of America
[3]School of Medicine, Copperbelt University, Ndola, Zambia
[4]University of Lusaka, Lusaka, Zambia

Arthropod-borne viruses (arboviruses) have become significant public health problems, with the emergency and re-emergency of arboviral diseases nearly worldwide. The objective of this study was to determine the prevalence and the risk factors for Zika virus infection in North-Western Province of Zambia.

* Correspondence: Peter Songolo, MBChB, MPH, World Health Organization, Lusaka, Zambia. E-mail: songolop@who.int.

A cross-sectional study using a standardised questionnaire was used. Bivariate logistic regression analyses were conducted to obtain odds ratios and their 95% confidence intervals. In total, 1,755 survey participants were recruited. Overall, 48.8% of the survey participants were males. Males tended to have higher education levels than females, with 37.4% of males and 26.0% of females having attained secondary or higher levels of education ($p<0.001$). Altogether, 1.8% of participants had Zika virus infection, with no sex difference (2.1% of males and 1.4% of females, $p=0.957$). Visiting Angola was the only factor that was significantly associated with Zika virus infection. Participants who visited Angola were 2.82 (95% CI [1.82, 4.38]) times more likely to have Zika virus infection compared to participants who had not visited Angola. Zika virus infection is prevalent among residents of North-Western Province in Zambia. Strengthening of disease surveillance, clinical management of cases and laboratory diagnostic capacities are necessary to curb the infection.

INTRODUCTION

Zambia is undergoing rapid developmental changes particularly in infrastructure. The opening up of new mines in recent years in North-Western province means that mining has become a major occupation for the province. This has resulted in population movement especially from the 'traditional' Copperbelt province, creating a sudden increase in the total population of the province with resultant challenges for the health sector. Sudden population increase has resulted in over-crowding creating a suitable environment for disease spread including the arboviruses.

Among the emerging infectious diseases, the arboviral diseases group has particularly warranted attention in the global health landscape with its potential for epidemics and its unprecedented spread (1). Despite the significance and increasing public health impact on individuals worldwide, arboviruses remain poorly understood and controlled. While increasingly well characterised in industrialised countries, the epidemiology of the these viruses is a major challenge to developing countries and surveillance often is usually in the form of reports during outbreaks due to the poor population-based surveillance systems (2). The majority of the surveillance systems were designed to detect known pathogens (61.5%), while 19.9% were for both known and unknown pathogens and only a small proportion were designed to detect unknown pathogens (3).

The diagnosis of Zika virus infection is based on detection of specific antibodies (4) or virus isolation from animals or mosquitoes which is time consuming; however, rapid diagnostic methods have been developed for the African and Asian strains (5). Several serological surveys have been carried out in Africa and notable among these is the Portuguese Guinea survey which demonstrated frequent antibodies to group B viruses particularly Yellow Fever, Zika and Wesselbrons; a finding similar to previous surveys in the same region (6). Based on serological analyses, flaviviruses were classified into eight antigenic complexes; however, many viruses including the prototype of the group Yellow Fever and many new viruses could not be affiliated to any complex partly due to extensive geographical distribution, diversity of arthropod vector or vertebrate hosts and also confusion in virus nomenclature (7).

No information on Zika virus infection has been reported in Zambia. The objective of the study was, thus, to determine the prevalence and correlates for Zika virus infection in North-Western province of Zambia in order to contribute to the body of knowledge on the epidemiology of Zika virus infection in Zambia.

OUR STUDY

North-Western Province borders with Angola in the West and Democratic Republic of Congo (DRC) in the North. North-Western Province was one of Zambia's nine provinces at the time of the survey before the creation of the tenth province. It covers an area of 125,826 km^2 and had a population of 695,599 (8).

A total of 1,178 Standard Enumeration Areas (SEAs) were demarcated in North-Western province in the eight districts of the province. North-Western province is located in Agro-ecological zone III which is suitable for cultivating rice, cassava, pineapples and bananas (9).

The data was obtained from a survey on Yellow fever. The sample size calculation was based on the assumption that the sero-prevalence for Yellow fever was 7% based on the study conducted by Robinson (10). A Statcal program in Epi Info v6.04 was used to estimate the sample size. After adjusting for 80% response rate, a sample size of 3600 was obtained. The sample size was equally divided into the two provinces and powered to avoid chance findings, that is, 1,800 participants from each province.

A multi-stage sampling technique was used for participants in all districts. Firstly, wards were randomly selected from each constituency. In the second stage of sampling, standard enumeration areas (SEAs) proportional to the ward size were systematically sampled. All survey participants aged nine months or older in a selected household were eligible to be enrolled in the study.

The study protocol was reviewed and approved by the Tropical Diseases Research Centre Research Ethics Committee, and permission to conduct the study was obtained from the Ministry of Health, Zambia. Informed consent was obtained from survey participants after the interviewer had explained the benefits and risks of participating in the study. Entry forms were viewed only by those approved to be part of the survey.

A detailed semi structured questionnaire was used to collect information. During the data collection process, questionnaires were checked for inconsistencies and completeness on a daily basis.

All data were entered in an Epi-Info data entry screen that had consistency and range checks embedded in it. Epi data files were exported to SPSS for data analysis. Further editing was conducted by running frequencies during the analysis stage. Odds ratios and their 95% confidence intervals were used to estimate magnitudes of associations.

OUR FINDINGS

In total, 1755 survey participants were recruited. Overall, 48.8% of the survey participants were males. Males tended to have higher education levels than females, with 37.4% of males and 26.0% of females having attained secondary or higher levels of education ($p<0.001$). Altogether, 1.8% of participants had Zika virus infection, with no sex difference (2.1% of males and 1.4% of females, $p=0.957$).

Visiting Angola was the only factor that was significantly associated with Zika virus infection. Participants who visited Angola were 2.82 (95% CI [1.82, 4.38]) times more likely to have Zika virus infection compared to participants who had not visited Angola. Age, sex, education, use of mosquito net and in-door residual spraying were not significantly associated with Zika virus infection.

Table 1. Sample description for North-Western Province for Zika virus infection

Factor	Total n (%)	Male n (%)	Female n (%)	p value
Age (years)				
< 15	533 (30.4)	267 (31.3)	265 (29.5)	0.102
15 – 24	348 (19.8)	164 (19.2)	182 (20.3)	
25 – 34	348 (19.8)	151 (17.7)	197 (22.0)	
35 – 44	247 (14.1)	121 (14.2)	125 (13.9)	
45+	278 (15.8)	150 (17.6)	128 (14.3)	
Sex				
Male	854 (48.8)			
Female	897 (51.2)			
Education				
None	370 (21.4)	160 (19.1)	209 (23.6)	<0.001
Primary	812 (47.0)	365 (43.5)	445 (50.3)	
Secondary or higher	545 (31.6)	314 (37.4)	230 (26.0)	
Zika virus infection				
Yes	31 (1.8)	18 (2.1)	13 (1.4)	0.957
No	1724 (98.2)	836 (97.9)	884 (98.6)	

Table 2. Factors associated with Zika virus infection in North-Western Province in bivariate logistic regression analysis

Factor	OR (95% CI)
Age (years)	
< 15	0.37 (0.14, 0.99)
15 – 24	0.38 (0.12, 1.21)
25 – 34	1.15 (0.54, 2.47)
35 – 44	1.19 (0.93, 3.96)
45+	1
Sex	
Male	1.21 (0.84, 1.73)
Female	1
Education	
None	0.82 (0.43, 1,58)
Primary	1.36 (0.84, 2.22)
Secondary or higher	1

Table 2. (Continued)

Factor	OR (95% CI)
Use of mosquito net	
Yes	1.27 (0.87, 1.86)
No	1
In-door residual spraying	
Yes	0.96 (0.64, 1.43)
No	1
Visited Angola	
Yes	2.82 (1.82, 4.38)
No	1

DISCUSSION

Information concerning the distribution of Zika virus in North-Western Province was non-available until after the risk assessment was conducted in April/May 2013 by the Ministry of Health with the support of World Health Organization. The risk assessment carried out in North-Western Province was conducted to respond to the re-classification of the province as a low-risk area for arboviruses particularly Yellow Fever. There was no assessment carried out in the province since 1950 when the last sero-survey was conducted during the colonial era. The sero-survey of 1950 concentrated in Barotseland (Western), Balovale (North-Western) and Ndola in present day Copperbelt Province (10).

Zika virus which had not been previously reported in North-Western Province appeared to be an important flavivirus affecting 1.8% of the survey participants. Our finding indicates that Zika virus was circulating among people of North-Western Province. Our finding is much lower than those reported in Kainji lake basin of Nigeria of 56% (11), Oyo State of Nigeria of 31% (12), Yap island of Federated States of Micronesia of 73% (13). Differences in rates of infection may partly be due to different laboratory tests, power of the studies and epidemiological stages of the infection in study areas.

The risk assessment revealed that international travel especially outside of the province was highly associated with acquisition of infection for Zika virus. The survey participants with a history of travel to neighbouring countries especially to the Republic of Angola had twice as much risk of acquiring Zika infection than their counterparts without history of travel. However, travel to the Democratic Republic of Congo was not found to be significant probably due to host ecology and host behaviour (14). Stoddard et al., using mathematical models, illustrated the importance of human movement in the transmission of pathogens especially for populations most at risk to vector-borne diseases such as Zika virus (15).

Despite the fact that 1.8% of samples collected during the risk assessment tested positive for Zika virus infection, no human case of Zika disease has been reported from North-Western Province. This may be due to the lack of knowledge by the medical personnel and also due to the absence of case definition in the Integrated Diseases Surveillance and Response (IDSR) guidelines which are widely used for syndromic diseases surveillance in health facilities. Furthermore, the symptoms of Zika infection apart from being sub-clinical in presentation could be mimicking malaria which has been known to be prevalent in the province. Therefore, suspected malaria cases might have continued to mask outbreaks of Zika virus infection.

The other challenge contributing to lack of information on arboviral disease presence or absence is the limitation on availability of diagnostic methods, thereby making it difficult to identify these emerging diseases in the country. Until 2013 in preparation for the risk assessment on Yellow Fever, the laboratory capacity to diagnose arboviruses had not been developed.

In conclusion, Zika virus infection is prevalent among residents of North-Western Province in Zambia. Strengthening of disease surveillance, clinical management of cases and laboratory diagnostic capacities are necessary to curb the infection.

ACKNOWLEDGMENTS

We are grateful to the interviewers for their dedicated work to successfully complete the survey. The survey could not have been successful without the cooperation of the participants and the virology laboratory staff both in Lusaka, Zambia and Dakar, Senegal for in testing samples. The survey was funded by the Ministry of Health [Zambia] and the World Health Organization.

REFERENCES

[1] Dash AP, Bhatia R, Sunyoto T, Mourya DT. Emerging and re-emerging arboviral diseases in South-East Asia. J Vector Borne Dis 2013;50:77-84.

[2] Kuniholm MK, Wolfe ND, Huang CYH, Mpoudi-Ngole E, Tamufe U, Burke DS, Duane J. Gubler DJ. Seroprevalence and distribution of Flaviviridae, Togaviridae and Bunyaviridae arboviral infection in rural Cameroonian adults. Am J Trop Med Hyg 2006;74:1078-83.

[3] Vrbova L, Stephen C, Kasman N, Boehnke R, Doyle-Waters M, Chablitt-Clark A, Gibson B, FitzGerald M, Patrick DM. Systematic review of surveillance systems for emerging zoonoses. Trandbound Emerg Dis 2010;57:154-61.

[4] Causey OR, Theiler M. Virus antibody survey on sera of residents of the Amazon valley in Brazil. Am J Trop Med Hyg 1958;7:36-41.

[5] Faye O, Faye O, Diallo D, Diallo M, Weidman M, Sall AA. Quantitative real-time PCR detection of Zika virus and evaluation with filed-caught mosquitoes. Virol J 2013;10:311.

[6] Pinto MR. Survey for antibodies to Arboviruses in the sera of children in Portuguese Guinea. Bull World Hlth Org 1967;37:101-8.

[7] Kuno G, Chang GJ, Tsuchiya KR, Kabaratsos N, Cropp CB. Phylogeny of the genus flaviviruses. J Virol 1998;72:73-83.

[8] Central Statistical Office. 2010 census of population and housing. National analytical report. Lusaka, Zambia: CSO, 2012.

[9] Country profile-Zambia. New Agriculturist. Accessed 2014 May 19. URL: http://www.new-ag.info/en/country/profile.php?a=2621.

[10] Robinson GG. A note on mosquitoes and yellow fever in Northern Rhodesia. East Afr Med J 1950;27:284-8.

[11] Adekolu-John EO, Fagbami AH. Arthropod-borne virus antibodies in sera of rfesidents of Kainji lake basin, Nigeria 1980. Trans R Soc Trop Med Hyg 1983;77:149-51.

[12] Fagbami AH. Zika virus infections in Nigeria: virological and seroepidemiological investigations in Oyo State. J Hyg (Camb) 1979;83:213-9.

[13] Duffy MR, Chen T-H, Hancock TW, Powers AM, Kool JL, Lanciotti RS, Pretrick M, Marfel M, Holzbauer S, Dubray C, Guillaumot L, Griggs A, Bel M, Lambert AJ, Laven J, Kosoy O, Panella A, Biggerstaff BJ, Fischer M, Hayes EB. Zika virus outbreak on Yap island, Federated States of Micronesia. N Eng J Med 2009;360:2536-43.

[14] Reiter P. Climate change and mosquito-borne disease: knowing the horse before hitching the cart. Rev Sci Tech Off Int 2008;27:383-98.

[15] Stoddard ST, Morrison AC, Vazquez-Prokopec GM, Soldan VP, Kochel TJ, Kitron U, Elder JP, Scott TW. The role of human movement in the transmission of vector-borne pathogens. PLoS PLoS Negl Trop Dis 2009;3:e481.

In: Arbovirus
Editors: S. Siziya, M. L. Mazaba et al.
ISBN: 978-1-63463-601-8

Chapter 6

RISK FOR WEST NILE VIRUS INFECTION

Idah Mweene-Ndumba, BSc, MPH[1,3*],
Seter Siziya, BA(Ed), MSc, PhD[2],
Mwaka Monze, MBhB, PhD[3],
Mazyanga L Mazaba, BSc, MSc[1,3],
Freddie Masaninga, BSc, MSc, PhD[1],
Peter Songolo, MBChB, MPH[1],
Peter Mwaba, MBChB, PhD[4],
and Olusegun Babaniyi, MBBS, MPH, MSc[1]
[1]World Health Organization, Lusaka, Zambia, [2]School of Medicine, Copperbelt University, Ndola, Zambia/University of Lusaka, Lusaka, Zambia, [3]University Teaching Hospital, Lusaka, Zambia, [4]Ministry of Home Affairs, Lusaka, Zambia

West Nile virus infection has been reported in Asia, Middle East, Europe, Americas and Africa but there is no documentation about its existence in Zambia. Therefore the purpose of this study was to determine the seroprevalence of WNV infection and its correlates in North-Western province of Zambia. Secondary data collected in a yellow fever risk assessment conducted in Zambia in 2013 was used in this study. Bivariate and

[*] Correspondence: Idah Mweene-Ndumba, BSc, MPH, World Health Organization, Lusaka, Zambia. E-mail: idahndumba12@gmail.com.

multivariate logistic regression analyses were used to determine correlates for WNV infection. Unadjusted odds ratios and adjusted odds ratios with their 95% Confidence Intervals (CI) are reported. Out of a total of 1,755 participants in the survey, 51.3% were females. About a third of the participants (30%) were aged 5 -14 years. Overall, 2.0% of the participants had WNV infection. Having travelled to Angola was independently associated with WNV infection. Participants who visited Angola were 2.58 (95% CI [1.67, 3.98]) times more likely to have WNV infection compared to those who had not travelled to Angola. Instituting an active surveillance for the infection at border post would help in preventing further importation of the virus.

INTRODUCTION

West Nile virus (WNV) is an arthropod borne virus from the Flaviviridae family. Humans get infected from a *culex* mosquito bite. Most of the infections are asymptomatic but about 1% show symptoms which sometimes could develop into severe illness (nueroinvasive symptoms) which could also result into death (1).

West Nile fever was first identified in a woman from the west Nile province, Uganda, who presented with influenza like illness in Uganda (2). After the discovery in Uganda the virus became endemic in many African countries, mainly epizootic at that time, with reported seasonal outbreaks in humans (3). The disease was viewed as of very low public health importance till its recognition as an emerging infectious disease as it spread across the globe with reports in Asia, Middle East, Europe and Americas (4-6). In North Africa, a more virulent strain of WNV emerged in 1994 and it caused outbreaks of severe disease symptoms and more deaths than reported previously (5).

Several risk factors for WNV infection emerged from the study in America such as climate and environmental factors. High population density was significantly associated with the viral transmission even after adjusting for other environmental factors (7) and the results were comparable to results obtained in other studies which confirmed an association between urban/sub-urban versus a more rural area (8,9). However other studies reported significant association when there was less population density and rural. Temperature changes determining human activity and mosquito replication was also significantly associated with risk of infection. It was also concluded that these factors could differ yearly due to changes in bird populations with high bird population as being protective (7). It is possible that when there are more birds the virus could be concentrated in bird mosquito bird cycle whereas if there are fewer birds the mosquito could resort to human meals. Studies have also confirmed that age has a bearing on the severity of the infection with the older age group, 50 years and above, being most at risk (7). In Arizon staying at home and not attending school were found to be risk factors to the WNV infection, although it was argued that the possibility that those who stayed at home were the elderly who were already known to be at high risk of infection with WNV (10).

Although WNV infections have been reported worldwide and furthermore around Zambia's neighboring countries, there is still no information on the extent of the problem in the North-western province of Zambia. Therefore the purpose of this analysis was to determine the seroprevalence of WNV and its correlates in North-western province of Zambia.

OUR STUDY

The study was conducted in North-Western province of Zambia. The province was selected based on the classification as low potential risk area for yellow fever transmission by World Health Organization (11). North-Western province, which borders with Angola on the western side and Democratic Republic of Congo (DRC) on the northern side, has a population of 706,462 (12). It is the most sparsely populated province in the country and the provincial capital is Solwezi. The province comprised of 8 districts which were divided into 1178 Standard Enumeration Aras (SEAs) and the main economic activities were mining in one district and general pineapple growing.

Study population, sample size, inclusion/exclusion criteria and sampling

This assessment was carried out among individuals aged nine months or older. In estimating the sample size for persons aged 5 years or older, the following parameters were considered: a prevalence of 7% (13), desired precision or confidence interval (d) of $\pm$3%, and a design effect (DE) of 2 and an 80% response rate.

Table 1. Sample description North-Western province

Factors	Total n (%)	Male n (%)	Female n (%)	P value
Age (years)				
5-14	533 (30.4)	267 (31.3)	265 (29.5)	0.102
15-24	348 (19.8)	164 (19.2)	182 (20.3)	
25-34	348 (19.8)	151 (17.7)	197 (22.0)	
25-44	247 (14.1)	121 (14.2)	125 (13.9)	
45+	278 (15.8)	150 (17.6)	128 (14.3)	
Sex				
Male	854 (48.8)	-	-	-
Female	897 (51.2)	-	-	
Education				
None	370 (21.4)	160 (19.1)	209 (23.6)	<0.001
Primary	812 (47.0)	365 (43.5)	445 (50.3)	
Secondary/College/ University	545 (31.6)	314 (37.4)	230 (26.0)	
West Nile Infection				
Positive	35 (2.0)	19 (2.2)	16 (1.8)	0.625
Negative	1720 (98.0)	835 (97.8)	881 (98.2)	

Considering sex, we aimed to recruit 700 male and 700 female participants in each province. Assuming an average of 4 persons aged 5 years or older in each household, a total of 12 households in each of the 30 cluster was to be recruited in the survey. The total number of persons that would be recruited from each province was 1806, totaling 3612 from both provinces.

The sero-prevalence of children was about half that for older children, and in estimating the sample size for persons aged below 5 years, the following parameters were considered: a prevalence of 3.5%, desired precision or confidence interval (d) of +3.4%, and a design effect (DE) of 2 and an 80% response rate. The computed sample size was 282. Therefore, in each province 406 children would be recruited for the survey.

Included in the study were individuals aged 9 months or older who were found in a sampled household at the time of the study and were resident in the study site for at least seven days. Individuals who had received YF vaccination in the last ten years to the survey were also included in the survey. Excluded from the study were persons who were aged less than 9 months, or individuals regardless of age who resided in the study site for less than 7 days prior to the survey. Children under the age of 9 months were excluded based on the fact that at this age children could still carry maternal antibodies from exposed mothers which could pose the risk of false positive results.

The sample was drawn using a two-stage cluster sampling technique using probability proportional to size. A list of the standard enumeration areas (SEAs) in each province constituted the sampling frame. The sampling was designed to achieve fairly good estimates at the provincial level of analysis, and not representing the subdivisions of the province.

Study variables

Dependent variable

A case with evidence of WNV exposure was defined as any individual aged 9 months or older whose blood sample was confirmed to have WNV exposure. WNV exposure status was positive if IgG or IgM antibodies were determined in the serum sample by laboratory testing and negative if the IgG or IgM antibodies were absent by laboratory testing.

Independent variables

The independent variables included demographic data: age, sex, occupation, education, roof type and use of mosquito preventive measures such as insecticide treated nets (ITNs) and indoor residual spray (IRS).

Laboratory procedures

Three to 5 millilitres of blood was collected by venepuncture into an EDTA vaccutainer tube and transported on cold chain to the local laboratories for serum separation and storage.

Subsequently serum samples were transported on cold chain and thereafter subjected to primary testing (YFV specific IgG and IgM) at the University of Teaching Hospital in Zambia virology unit and Institute Pasteur, Dakar. All presumptive YFV-specific IgG and IgM samples were subjected to IgG and IgM antibodies testing against other flaviviruses known to cause haemorrhagic fever-like disease including WNV. The testing was carried out using IgG capture enzyme-linked immunosorbent assay (ELISA).

Data management and analysis

Data collected from the field were entered in an Epi-Info data entry screen that had consistency and range checks embedded in it. Further editing was conducted by running frequencies during the analysis stage. Epi data files were exported to SPSS for data analysis. The data was summarized to describe the occurrence of WNV exposed individuals in absolute numbers and percentage by place (residence, travel or work) and person (age, sex, occupation, education). Further analysis was conducted to determine independent factors associated with WNV sero-positivity. Odds ratios were used to estimate the magnitude of associations.

Ethical considerations

Ethical clearance was sought from the Tropical Diseases Research Centre Research Ethics Committee, and ethical standards were adhered to throughout this study. Informed consent was sought from study participants. Guardians provided assent for the participation of the persons under the consenting age. They were asked to read or have read to them, understand and sign/thumbprint an informed consent form. Responsible adults in the household were identified to give proxy consent on behalf of minors.

OUR FINDINGS

Out of a total of 1755 participants in the survey, 51.3% were females. Most of the participants (30%) were aged 5 -14 years of age. There were more females who had attained primary school than males (p=0.001). On the other hand more males (37.4% males and 26% females) attained secondary or higher education than the females. There was no significant association between WNV infection and sex (p=0.625). Overall, 2.0% of the participants had antibodies to WNV.

The variables in Table 2, age, sex, education, sleeping under a mosquito net, house with IRS and travelled to Angola were analyzed in bivariate and multivariate models. Having travelled to Angola was the only factor that was significantly associated with WNV infection in multivariate analysis. Participants who visited Angola were 2.58 (95% CI [1.67, 3.98]) times more likely to have WNV infection compared with those who had not travelled to Angola.

Table 2. Factors associated with West Nile Virus infection in bivariate and multivariate analysis for North-Western province

Factor	OR (95% CI)	AOR (95% CI)
Age (years)		
5-14	0.59 (0.29-1.21)	-
15-24	0.45 (0.17-1.17)	
25-34	0.91 (0.44-1.87)	
35-44	1.96 (1.04-3.69)	
45+	1	
Sex		
Male	1.12 (0.80-1.57))	-
Female	1	
Education		
None	0.74 (0.39-1.40)	-
Primary	1.36 (0.85-2.16)	
Secondary/College/University	1	
Slept under mosquito net		
Yes	1.30 (0.90-1.86)	-
No	1	
House with IRS		
Yes	1.41 (1.01-1.99)	-
No	1	
Travelled to Angola		
Yes	2.61 (1.69-4.02)	2.58 (1.67-3.98)
No	1	1

DISCUSSION

This study presents the first documentation of the prevalence of WNV infection and the contributing factors to the infection in North-western province of Zambia This study has indicated that 2.0% of the participants had antibodies to WNV. This finding is similar to a 2.6% reported in New York during the 1999 epidemic (14), implying that both epidemics might have been at the same stage of the epidemic. A study conducted in Kenya reported varying rates of the infection of 3.2-65.3% within the same country (15). Higher rates of the infection have been reported in Egypt and Sudan of 61% and 40%, respectively (16) and 55% in South Africa (17) as way back as the 1950s to 1970s. Disease prevalence is dependent upon a wide range of risk factors, climate and the environment affecting the activities of the virus and the humans (7, 8, 9). It is therefore important that surveys be conducted not only in specific regions of a country but the whole country in order to inform the designs of interventions to curtail the spread of the virus.

Travelling to Angola was associated with being infected with WNV. Travel could have been necessitated by visiting relatives across the border in Angola or to conduct trade. While in Angola, one could have been bitten by an infected mosquito. A similar observation was made by Cameron et al. who observed that the continued spread of dengue was supported by global trade and increasing travel within and between countries (18). Furthermore, travel increases the risk of introducing arthropod-borne virus diseases from endemic to non-endemic areas.

In conclusion, surveillance at the border should be strengthened in order to curtail further importation of the virus into the province, assuming that persons who had traveled to Angola did not have the virus before they traveled.

ACKNOWLEDGMENTS

We are grateful to the interviewers for their dedicated work to successfully complete the survey. The survey could not have been successful without the cooperation of the participants and the virology laboratory staff both in Dakar, Senegal and Lusaka, Zambia for testing the samples. The survey was funded by the Ministry of Health [Zambia] and the World Health Organization.

REFERENCE

[1] Smithburn KC, Hughes TP, Burke AW, Paul JH. A neurotropic virus isolated from the blood of a native of Uganda. Am J Trop Med 1940;20:471-2.

[2] Petersen LR, Carson PJ, Biggerstaff BJ, Custer B, Borchardt SM, Busch MP. Estimated cumulative incidence of West Nile virus infection in US adults, 1999–2010. Epidemiol infect 2013;141(03): 591-5.

[3] Stiasny K, Aberle SW, HeinzFX. Retrospective identification of human cases of West Nile virus infection in Austria (2009 to 2010) by serological differentiation from Usutu and other flavivirus infections. Euro Surveill 2013;18(43). Pii:20614.

[4] Gubler DJ. The continuing spread of West Nile virus in the western hemisphere. Clin Infect Dis 2007;45:1039-46.

[5] Hayes EB, Komar N, Nasci RS, Montgomery SP, O'Leary DR, Campbell GL. Epidemiology and transmission dynamics of West Nile virus disease. Emerg Infect Dis 2005;11:1167-73.

[6] Liu A, Lee V, Galusha D, Slade MD, Diuk-Wasser M, Andreadis T, Scotch M, Rabinowitz PM. Risk factors for human infection with West Nile Virus in Connecticut: a multi-year analysis. Int J Health Geogr 2009;8:67.

[7] Brown HE, Childs JE, Diuk-Wasser MA, Fish D. Ecological factors associated with West Nile virus transmission, northeastern United States. Emerg Infect Dis 2008;14:1539-45.

[8] Gibbs SEJ, Wimberly MC, Madden M, Masour J, Yabsley MJ, Stallknecht DE. Factors Affecting the Geographic Distribution of West Nile Virus in Georgia, USA: 2002–2004. **Vector Borne** Zoonotic Dis 2006;6: 73-82.

[9] Gibney KB, Colborn J, Baty S, Bunko Patterson AM, Sylvester T, Briggs G, Stewart T, Levy C, Komatsu K, MacMillan K, Delorey MJ, Mutebi JP, Fischer M, Staples JE. Modifiable Risk Factors for West Nile Virus Infection during an Outbreak—Arizona, 2010. Am J Trop Med Hyg 2012;86:895–901.

[10] Schweitzer BK, Kramer WL, Sambol AR, Meza JL, Hinrichs SH, Iwen PC. Geographic Factors Contributing to a High Seroprevalence of West Nile Virus-Specific Antibodies in Humans following an Epidemic. Clin Vaccine Immunol 2006;13:314-8.

[11] Jentes ES, Poumerol G, Gershman MD, Hill DR, Lemarchand J, Lewis RF, Staples JE, Tomori O, Wilder-Smith A, Monath TP; Informal WHO Working Group on Geographic Risk for Yellow Fever. The revised global yellow fever risk map and recommendations for vaccination, 2010: consensus of the Informal WHO Working Group on Geographic Risk for Yellow Fever. Lancet Infect Dis 2011;11:622-32.

[12] Central Statistical Office. 2010 census of population and housing. National analytical report. Lusaka, Zambia: CSO, 2012

[13] Robinson GG. A note on mosquitoes and yellow fever in Northern Rhodesia. East Afr Med J 1950;27:284-8.

[14] Mostashari F, Bunning ML, Kitsutani PT, Singer DA, Nash D, Cooper MJ, Katz N, Liljebjelke KA, Biggerstaff BJ, Fine AD, Layton MC, Mullin SM, Johnson AJ, Martin DA, Hayes EB, Campbell GL. Epidemic West Nile encephalitis, New York, 1999: results of a household-based seroepidemiological survey. Lancet. 2001;358:261-4.

[15] Geser A, Henderson BE, Christensen S. A multipurpose serological survey in Kenya: 2. Results of arbovirus serological tests. Bull Wld Hlth Org 1970;43:539-52.

[16] Taylor RM, Work TH, Hurlbut HS, Rizk F. A study of the ecology of West Nile in Egypt. Am J Trop Med Hyg 1956;5:579-620.

[17] Mcintosh BM, Jupp PG, Dos Santos I, Meenehan GM. Epidemics of West Nile and Sindbis viruses in South Africa with Culex (Culex) univittatus Theobald as vector. South Afr J Sci 1976;72:295-300.

[18] Cameron P. Simmons CP, Farrar JJ, van Vinh Chau N, Wills B. Dengue. N Engl J Med 2012;366:1423-32.

In: Arbovirus
Editors: S. Siziya, M. L. Mazaba et al.
ISBN: 978-1-63463-601-8

Chapter 7

LARVAL HABITAT DISTRIBUTION: AEDES MOSQUITO VECTOR FOR ARBOVIRUSES AND CULEX SPPS

Freddie Masaninga, BSc, MSc, PhD*[*1],
Mbanga Muleba, BSc, MSc[2],
Hieronymo Masendu, BSc, MSc, PhD[3],
Peter Songolo, MBChB, MPH[1],
Idah Mweene-Ndumba, BSc, MPH[1],
Mazyanga L Mazaba, BSc, MSc[1],
Mulakwa Kamuliwo, MD[6],
Birknesh Ameneshewa, BSc, MSc, PhD[5],
Seter Siziya, BA(Ed), MSc, PhD[4],
and Olusegun A Babaniyi, MBBS, MPH, MSc[1]
[1]World Health Organization, Lusaka, Zambia, [2]Tropical Diseases Research Centre, Ndola, Zambia, [3]Abt Associates Harare, Zimbabwe, [4]The Copperbelt University, School of Medicine, Zambia/University of Lusaka, Lusaka, Zambia, [5]World Health Organization, Harare, Zimbabwe, [6]Ministry of Health, Lusaka, Zambia

[*] Correspondence: Freddie Masaninga, PhD, National Professional Officer, WHO Country Office, Lusaka, Zambia. E-mail: Masaningaf@who.int.

Zambia is prone to mosquito-borne diseases: malaria, filariasis and arthropod-borne viruses (arboviruses). There is limited information on the distribution of larval habitats of vectors of arboviruses in Zambia. A study was conducted to determine the distribution of mosquito larval habitats in Western and North-Western provinces of Zambia. Mosquito larval surveys were conducted in rural, urban and peri-urban locations, indoor and outdoor. Altogether, 350 potential breeding habitats were inspected: flower pots, old tires, banana leaf axils, water storage containers, shallow wells, disused wells, disused bottles, canoes and water pools soaked with cassava tubers. Aedes (stegomyia) aegypti larvae were collected in a disused cooking oil plastic container; 1 (1.9%) out of 52 containers in peri-urban areas of North-Western province was positive for larvae, while no container in Western province was positive for larvae. Culex quiquefasciatus larvae were collected in 12 (3.9%) of 350 containers outdoor in peri-urban, urban and rural areas, in abandoned water wells, discarded plastic containers, canoes and in water pools for processing cassava. Distribution of micro-habitats including those less suspected to be mosquito larval habitats by local communities highlights a need for strengthening vector surveillance to provide real-time entomological data for policy decisions.

INTRODUCTION

Mosquitoes transmit various mosquito-borne diseases such as malaria, filariasis and arthropod-borne viruses (arboviruses) including, dengue virus, yellow fever virus, West Nile virus and Zika virus (1-8). Zambia is prone to mosquito-borne diseases because it has suitable ecological and climatic conditions for mosquito vector survival throughout the year during the rainy and hot season (November-May) and cool dry season (June-September) (9, 10).

A yellow fever risk assessment survey (11) necessitated a similar entomological survey to obtain a greater understanding on the vector-larval distribution in relation to human settlements. Information on mosquito spatial distribution patterns in Zambia is limited and yet, its use could optimize resource utilization and hopefully contribute towards evidence-based vector control to reduce mosquito-borne diseases (12).

Mosquito breeding sites, areas where immature forms of mosquitoes transform and grow into the adult stage, are an important determinant of the distribution and abundance of adult forms of mosquitoes. Mosquito breeding habitats include containers for species such as Aedes aegypti, pit-latrines, waste water near human habitation for Culex quiquefasciatus mosquitoes and sunlit water pools for Anopheles mosquitoes. Removal of these sources would complement interventions that target adult forms of mosquitoes (13). Regular application of chemical and biological insecticides to malaria mosquito breeding sites, larviciding, is recommended where the sites are few, fixed and findable (14).

Accurate understanding of bionomics, distribution and seasonal changes of mosquito breeding habitats is vital for designing effective interventions for reducing mosquito population. While adult mosquito studies mainly on malaria vectors have been conducted (15), larval habitat distribution of Aedes mosquito vector for arboviruses is limited in Zambia. Therefore, an entomological survey was undertaken to determine the distribution of peridomestic larval breeding habitats for mosquito vectors of arboviruses in North-Western and Western provinces of Zambia bordering countries where arboviruses have been recently reported.

OUR STUDY

North-Western province is located at 1,354 metres above sea level, latitude -13.0 and longitude 25.0 and has a population of 706,462. The province borders with Angola on the western side and Democratic Republic of Congo on the northern side with population movement between countries. It has six districts at the time of the survey. The province receives the highest rainfall in the country, with annual rainfall of 1320 mm. The mean minimum temperature in June and mean maximum temperature in October are 6.8°C and 30.6°C, respectively (16). North-Western province is located within the Central African plateau. Rice, cassava, banana and pineapple cultivation is the main economic activity of the province.

Western province which borders with Angola has a population of 881,524 and had seven districts at the time of the survey (16). It is the driest area of Zambia and located at 1,119 metres above sea level and latitude -15.0 and longitude 24.0. The mean minimum and maximum temperatures of 8.7°C and 34.2°C are in June and October, respectively, and an annual rainfall of 740 mm (17). Western province major valleys extend to the Kalahari sand plateau and lies within the Zambezi flood plains. Crop and livestock production as well as fishing along the available water bodies are the main economic activities in the province.

Rural and urban or peri-urban areas: Classification into rural, urban and peri-urban was based on an analysis by the Department for International Development (DFID) of the United Kingdom, which took into account several parameters including access to basic services-health, education (and other social services) and population density (18).

Household: The term household as used in this study means one or more people who live in the same dwelling and also share meals or living accommodation (19).

Districts sampled

Mosquito sampling – larval and adult sampling were undertaken in North-Western province (Mwinilunga, Mufumbwe, Kabompo, Chavuma, Solwezi and Zambezi districts) and in Western province (in Kaoma and Mongu districts) of Zambia.

Training

Training in field mosquito larval sampling was conducted for a week at the Tropical Diseases Research Center, Ndola, Zambia and was facilitated by experts from the World Health Organization and Pasteur Institute, Dakar, Senegal. The training included larval sampling methods, preservation of entomological specimens and rearing of larvae to adults to enable identification of emerged adult mosquitos. The training helped to standardize the collection, preservation and analysis of the mosquito larval samples.

Mosquito larval sampling

Three teams of 3-4 research members undertook mosquito larval searches in rural, urban and peri-urban areas of the two provinces (North-Western and Western provinces) of Zambia. The target was to sample mosquito larvae inside and outside houses for each household visited covering at least 10 households per day. All containers kept inside houses were inspected for mosquito larvae (flower-pots and water storage). The following habitats outside houses were inspected: shallow wells, discarded clay-pots, discarded bottles, plastics containers, tyres, banana (Musa sapientum) leaf axils and edges of water canals. A larval scoop was used to collect water for larval inspection on a white tray. The collected mosquito larvae were pipetted and transferred into a bottle labeled with relevant information for identification such as province, district, locality (urban or rural), house number (randomly allocated during sampling), number of habitation units or occupied rooms and date of collection.

Types and characteristics of containers

Information was collected for each breeding habitat where mosquito larvae were collected. The information included type of breeding habitat and its purpose (whether for storage of drinking water or disused/discarded); whether breeding habitat was man-made (plastic containers, bottles, metal buckets, earthen pots, tyres or cement blocks) or natural (such as banana leaf axils and stagnant water pools); presence or absence of plant growth or debris inside or around container habitats; and latitude and longitude which were obtained using a Global Positioning System.

Distribution of larval habitats

To understand the distribution of the mosquito larval sites, different locations were searched in diverse potential mosquito breeding sites in urban and rural areas. The container index (CI) was estimated as percentage of containers found with mosquito larvae to determine the presence of disease-causing mosquitoes. A CI above 10% was considered high and this was the threshold that was used in this study. In the field, adult mosquitoes that emerged from pupae were cryopreserved in liquid nitrogen. Each cryo-tube was labeled with a unique code indicating household number and cluster number where larvae were collected in addition to the province and district codes.

Mosquito larval rearing

Sampled mosquito larvae were transported to the Tropical Diseases Research Centre insectary laboratory in Ndola, Zambia and bred through to the adult stage for species identification using entomological keys (20-22). Larvae were fed on fish flakes Tetramin and maintained at relative humidity of $80 \pm 2\%$ and temperature of 23±2°C. All emerged adult mosquitoes were stored at -80°C to preserve their viability prior to airfreighting them to Institute Pasteur in Dakar, Senegal for species identification.

Ethical considerations

Oral informed consent was obtained from heads of households in which larval inspections were undertaken. Written informed consent was obtained from all team members and local personnel who were involved in rearing mosquitoes.

Data analysis

Data were entered into Microsoft Excel 2010, checked for consistency and exported into SPSS version 16.0 for analysis.

OUR FINDINGS

Distribution of mosquito larvae habitats: The distribution of mosquito breeding habitats for Aedes species and Culex species in the North-Western and Western provinces are displayed in Tables 1 and 2, respectively. A total of 350 containers that were found indoor and outdoor were examined for mosquito larvae.

Types and characteristic of containers: A plastic container was the favoured breeding microhabitat for Aedes aegypti, with a density of at least 15 per larval scoop. Meanwhile, habitats for Culex quiquefasciatus larvae were abandoned water wells, shallow wells and canoes that contained a lot of organic matter. The canoes were overgrown with grass and plant vegetation.

Distribution of Aedes larvae: Aedes (stegomyia) aegypti larvae were collected in a dis-used cooking oil plastic container. One (1.9%) of the 52 containers in peri-urban locality of North-Western province was positive for larvae and none of the containers in Western province was positive for larvae. This discarded plastic container was located at the edge of a village. Aedes larvae were not collected in other habitats such as banana leaf axils, flower pots, cement blocks for house construction and discarded bottles.

Table 1. Distribution of Aedes species mosquito larvae in North Western and Western provinces, Zambia and percentage of containers positive for larvae, April-May, 2013

	No. Houses	Occupied rooms	Number of containers pos/exam Indoor [1]	pos/exam Outdoor [2]	%
North Western					
Peri-Urban	48	277	0/0	1/52	1.9
Urban	24	112	0/0	0/40	0.0
Rural	48	237	0/0	0/98	0.0
Western					
Urban	60	316	0/0	0/117	0.0
Rural	36	171	0/0	0/43	0.0

Indoor[1] containers were drinking-water-storage containers; outdoor[2] containers were flowerpots, discarded plastic, container and shallow wells; pos=positive; exam=examined.

Table 2. Distribution of *Culex* species mosquito larval stages in rural, urban and peri-urban areas of North Western and Western provinces of Zambia – April-May, 2013

Location	No. of Houses	occupied rooms	Number of containers Positive /Inspected	%
Peri-urban	48	277	6/64	9.4
Urban	84	428	3/174	1.7
Rural	84	408	3/112	2.6
Total				12/350

Distribution of Culex larvae: Culex quiquefasciatus larvae were collected in 12 (3.9%) of the 350 container habitats outdoor in peri-urban, urban and rural areas, in abandoned water wells, water pools and in discarded plastic containers. In North-Western province, Culex quiquefasciatus was also collected in water pools-soaked with cassava tuber to soften it prior to its pounding. The water pool was situated at a forested edge of a village (Figure 1). Culex quiquefasciatus larvae was also found in disused canoes containing wood fibre to soften it prior to use in house construction (Figure 2) and in Clay-pots (see figure 3).

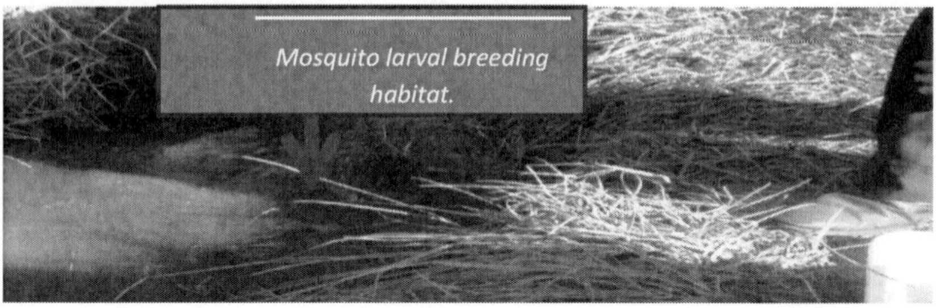

Figure 1. Breeding sites of *Culex quiquefasciatus* larvae in water pools soaked with cassava tubers in North Western province, Zambia.

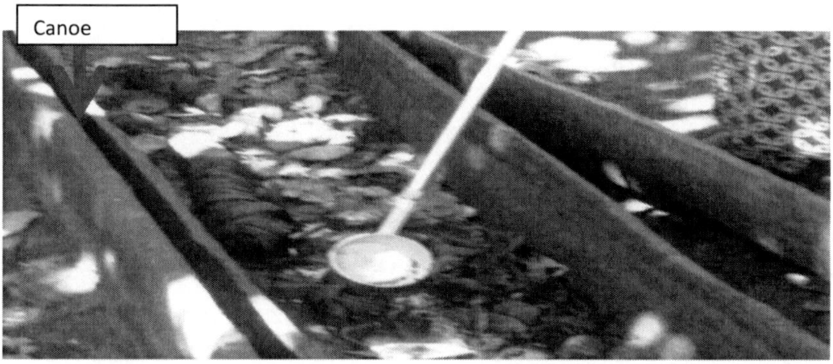

Figure 2. A canoe *Culex quiquefasciatus* was collected; this mosquito larval habitat contained wood fibre soaked in water to soften it before use. The position of the larval scoop (dipper) indicates the sites where the larvae were collected in Western Province of Zambia, Mongu District.

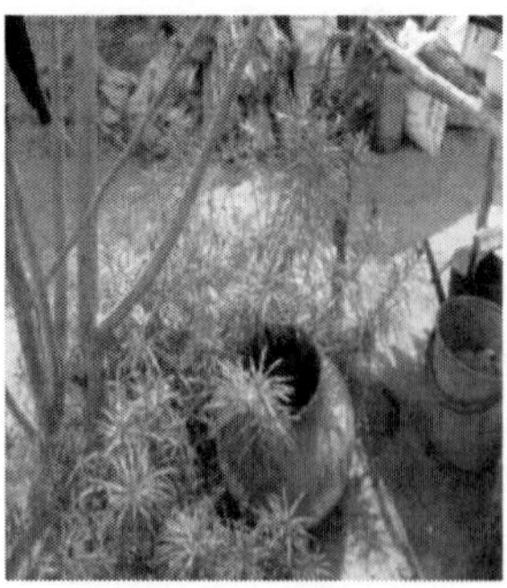

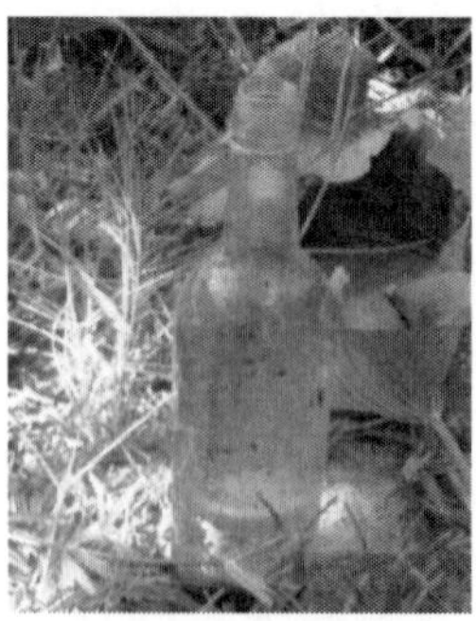

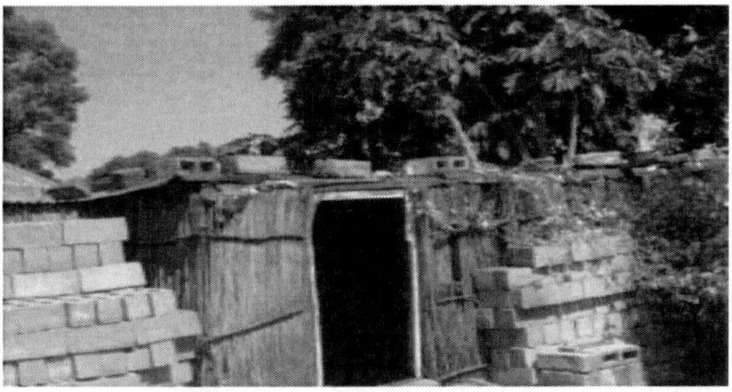

Figure 3. Various habitats searched for mosquito larva including clay pots, disused bottles, cement blocks placed by household owners to stop wind blowing roof tops, and cement blocks stored for future house construction.

Discussion

This study demonstrates Aedes mosquito larvae distribution in limited locations outdoor only in discarded plastic container in peri-urban areas of North-Western province of Zambia. No Aedes or other mosquito larval habitats were found indoor possibly since all water-storage containers were closed with a plastic cap. This is the first study in 64 years on Aedes bionomics during a yellow fever risk assessment survey in North-Western province. In the 1950s, Robinson (23) reported Aedes aegypti and Aedes africanus larvae breeding in tree holes during the wetter months of January-February in Baluvale location, currently called Zambezi, North-Western Province, Livingstone and Ndola. In those studies, only 1% of the 5,267 larvae collected was Aedes aegypti and 1% was Aedes africanus. In addition, Robinson observed that Aedes africanus was the commonest mosquito during the drier parts of the year (May-October). He found Aedes africanus breeding in bamboo (artificially made) pots in Ndola, Copperbelt, but rarely found Aedes aegypti and Aedes simpsoni larvae in other habitats that were searched (23). In addition, Robinson reported Aedes Aegypti larval habitats on rock pools in Livingstone. The finding of Aedes mosquito larvae in plastic containers corroborates the finding that was reported in a Nigerian study (24) which showed that the most preferred peri-domestic larval habitats were plastic containers (47%) followed by metal containers (35%) and earthen ware pots (14%). The plastic containers were mainly used by Aedes species, whereas earthen pots were mainly used by Anopheles species.

Table 3. Distribution of mosquito breeding sites by location and type of container in North Western and Western Province of Zambia April-May 2014

Location	Container	No. Positive/ Examined
Outdoor	Canoes	1/ 2
	Discarded plastic containers	2/ 67
	Discarded wells	2/ 8
	Flower pots	0/83
	Tyres	0/3
	Claypots	0/3
	Cement blocks	0/50
	Bottles (discarded)	0/1
	Banana leaf axils	0/27
	Water pools for soaking cassava	1/ 2
	Stagnant water pools	1/ 9
	Calabash	0/1
	Bucket water storage	0/20
Subtotal		**7/276**
Indoor	Bucket water storage	0/ 35
	Butiza (plastic) water storage	0/4
	Clay pot	0/1
	Plastic containers (Discarded)	0/34
Subtotal		**0/74**
Grand total		**7/350**

The Container Index (CI) reported in this study was 1.9% which is much lower than the 10% threshold above which is considered a problem in as far as yellow fever vector breeding is concerned. Recently, CI ranging from 38.7 to 79.3% have been reported during a yellow fever outbreak in central part of Senegal (25).

The presence of Aedes species in North-Western province and not in Western province despite having used similar sampling techniques could be explained by possible varying microhabitat, ecological and environmental conditions in the two provinces. North-Western province is wetter than

Western province, which is occupied by a large water body for approximately half of the year. Better adaptation of Aedes aegypti to arid conditions has been observed in a Cameroonian study but not in the current study (26).

This study demonstrates more diverse breeding habitats for Culex quiquefasciatus than Aedes. Culex quiquefasciatus larvae were collected in rural, urban and peri-urban locations. Some habitats such as water pools for cassava tubers were less suspected by the community for mosquito breeding. It was perceived that the environment created by the cassava tuber, with its possible cyanide and or/ fermentation products could present a less favorable microhabitat for larval breeding. This finding should be communicated to communities to enhance effective community-based integrated vector control. In a previous study we observed Culex quiquefasciatus mosquito larvae proliferating under water hyacinth in microhabitats located in sewer ponds which led to un precedent increased mosquito densities and biting, attesting further to the remarkable adaptation of Culex quiquefasciatus to different microhabitats (27).

Observations of Culex quiquefasciatus breeding in canoes that are used for soaking wood fibers for house construction calls for community health education on the role of various discarded containers and the activities that create conducive mosquito larval habitats. These observations underscore the increasing importance of Integrated Vector Management and the value of collaboration among researchers, policy makers in health and non-health and communities enshrined within an Integrated Vector Management concept to ensure a holistic approach in addressing challenges of vector control in public health (28, 29).

In conclusion, outdoor breeding habitats for Aedes (stegomyia) aegypti were limited but more abundant for Culex quiquefasciatus in all ecological locations (rural, urban and peri-urban) in water pools, canoes, discarded clay-pots and shallow water pool soaked with cassava. Continuous surveillance is essential to monitor breading sites for potential vectors for arbo-viruses to ensure evidenced-based interventions.

ACKNOWLEDGMENTS

We are grateful to heads of households for agreeing to survey both inside and outside their houses for mosquito larvae. The research assistants are thanked for their effort in making the survey a success. This study was funded by the

World health Organization and the Ministry of Health, Zambia as part of a yellow fever risk assessment survey in Zambia.

REFERENCES

[1] Rogers DJ, Wilson AJ, Hay SI, Graham AJ. The Global Distribution of Yellow Fever and Dengue. Adv Parasitol 2006;62:18-22.

[2] Mondet B, da Rosa AP, Vasconcelos PF. The risk of urban yellow fever outbreaks in Brazil by dengue vectors. Aedes aegypti and Aedes albopictus. Int J Infect Dis 2012;16:27.

[3] World Health Organisation (WHO). Wkly Epidemiol Rec 2013;88:201-16.

[4] Gubler DJ. The changing epidemiology of yellow fever and dengue, 1900 to 2003: full circle? Comp Immunol Microbiol Infect Dis 2004;27:319-30.

[5] Phoutrides EK, Coulibaly MB, George CM, Sacko A, Traore S, Bessoff K, et al. Dengue virus seroprevalence among febrile patients in Bamako, Mali: results of a 2006 surveillance study. Vector Borne Zoonotic Dis 2011;11:1479-85.

[6] De Filette M, Ulbert S, Diamond M, Sanders NN. Recent progress in West Nile virus diagnosis and vaccination. Vet Res 2012;43:16.

[7] Kautner I, Robinson MJ, Kuhnle U. Dengue virus infection: Epidemiology, pathogenesis, clinical presentation, diagnosis, and prevention. J Pediatr 1997;131:516-24.

[8] Grard G, Caron M, Mombo IM, Nkoghe D, Ondo SM, Jiolle D, et al. Zika Virus in Gabon (Central Africa) - 2007: A new threat from Aedes Albopictus? PLoS Negl Trop Dis 2014;8:1-6.

[9] Central Statistical Office. Zambia 2010 Census of population and housing. National Descriptive Tables. Lusaka, Central Statistical Office. Accessed 2014, August 27. URL; www.zamstats.gov.zm.

[10] Ministry of Health (MOH). Guidelines for Epidemic Preparedness, Prevention and Control of malaria in Zambia second Edition. Lusaka: Government Printers, 2007:3-13.

[11] Mazaba-Liwewe ML, Siziya S, Monze M, Mweene-Ndumba I, Masaninga F, Songolo P, et al. First sero-prevalence of dengue fever specific immunoglobulin G antibodies in Western and North-Western provinces of Zambia: a population based cross sectional study. Virol J 2014;11:135.

[12] Van den BH, Mutero CM, Ichimori K. Guidance on policy-making for Integrated Vector Management. Geneva: WHO, 2012.

[13] Orshan L, Bin H, Schnur H, Kaufman A, Valinsky A, Shulma L, et al. Mosquito Vectors of West Nile Fever in Israel. J Med Entomol 2008;45:939-47.

[14] WHO. The role of larviciding in sub-Saharan Africa. Interim Position Statement. Global Malaria Programme. Geneva: WHO, 2012.

[15] Masaninga F, Chanda E, Chanda-Kapata P, Hamainza B, Masendu HT, Kamuliwo M, et al. Review of the malaria epidemiology and trends in Zambia. Asian Pac J Trop Biomed 2013;3:89-94.

[16] Climate of Zambia. Accessed 2014 August 27. URL: http://www. zambiatourism. com/about-zambia/climate.

[17] Aregheore EM. Country Pasture/Forage Resource, Zambia. Accessed 2014 August 27. URL: http://www.fao.org/ag/AGP/AGPC/doc/Counprof/zambia/zambia. htm#_Toc131995463

[18] Department for International Development. Urban and rural change. Accessed 2014 August 27. URL: http://eldis.org/vfile/upload/1/document/0901/UR_overview.pdf.

[19] Zambia National Malaria Indicator Survey 2012. Government of the Republic of Zambia. Ministry of Health, Central Statistical Office, PATH, MACEPA, CDC, WHO. Accessed 2014 August 27. URL: http://www.nmcc.org.zm/files/FullReport ZambiaMIS2012_July2013_withsigs2.pdf.

[20] Gillies MT, Coetzee M. A supplement to the anophelinae of Africa South of the Sahara (Afrotropical Region). Johannesburg: Publications of the South African Institute for Medical Research, 1987.

[21] Rueda ML. Pictorial keys for the identification of mosquitoes (Diptera: Culicidae) associated with Dengue Virus Transmission. Auckland, New Zealand: Magnolia Press, 2004:14-22.

[22] Yiau-Min H. A pictorial key for the identification of the subfamilies of Culicidae, genera of Culicinae, and subgenera of Aedes mosquitoes of the Afrotropical region (Diptera: Culicidae). Proceedings of the Entomological Society of Washington 2001;103:1-53.

[23] Robinson GG. A Note on Mosquitoes and Yellow Fever in Northern Rhodesia. East Afr Med J 1950;27: 284-8.

[24] Okogun GRA, Nwoke BEB, Okere AN, Anosike JC, Esekhegbe AC. Epidemiological Implications of preferences of breeding sites of mosquito species in Midwestern Nigeria. Ann Agric Environ Med 2003;10:217–22.

[25] Diallo M, Tall A, Dia I, Ba Y, Sarr FD, Ly AB, et al. Yellow fever outbreak in central part of Senegal. Epidemiological findings. J Public Health Epidemiol 2013; 5:291-6.

[26] Kamgang B, Happi JY, Boisier P, Njokou F, Herve JP, Simard F, et al. Geographic and ecological distribution of Dengue and Chikungunya virus vectors of Aedes aegypti and Aedes albopictus in three major Cameroonian towns. Med Vet Entomol 2010;24:132-41.

[27] Masaninga F, Nkhuwa DCW, Goma FM, Shinondo C, Chanda E, Kamuliwo M, et al. Mosquito biting and malaria situation in an urban setting in Zambia. J Public Hlth Epidemiol 2012;4:261-9.

[28] Chanda E, Masaninga F, Coleman M, Sikaala C, Katebe C, MacDonald M, et al. Integrated vector management: The Zambian experience. Malar J 2008;7:164.

[29] Chanda E, Govere JM, Macdonald MB, Lako RL, Haque U, Baba SP, et al. Integrated vector management: a critical strategy for combating vector-borne diseases in South Sudan. Malar J 2013;12:369.

In: Arbovirus
Editors: S. Siziya, M. L. Mazaba et al.
ISBN: 978-1-63463-601-8

Chapter 8

RISK ASSESSMENT FOR YELLOW FEVER

Olusegun Babaniyi, MBBS, MPH, MSc[1*],
Mazyanga L Mazaba, BSc, MSc[1],
Freddie Masaninga, BSc, MSc, PhD[1],
Peter Mwaba, MBChB, MMed[2],
David Mulenga, BSc, MPH[3],
Peter Songolo, MBChB, MPH[1],
Idah Mweene-Ndumba, BSc, MPH[1],
Emmanuel Rudatsikira, MD, MPH, DrPH[4],
and Seter Siziya, BA(Ed), MSc, PhD[3]
[1]World Health Organization, Lusaka, Zambia
[2]Ministry of Home Affairs, Lusaka, Zambia
[3]School of Medicine, Copperbelt University, Ndola, Zambia
[4]School of Health Professions, Andrews University, Michigan, United States of America

Western province of Zambia was reclassified from a no risk to a low risk area for YF in 2010. To ascertain this reclassification, an assessment for the risk of YF was conducted in 2013. Altogether, 1824 persons participated in the survey of which 44.8% were males. Overall, 9 (0.5%) of the participants had YF virus infection. Of the 9 cases of YF, 6 were

* Correspondence: Olusegun A. Babaniyi, MBBS, MPH, MSc, World Health Organization, Lusaka, Zambia. E-mail: agbagba@yahoo.com.

males. The age range for the cases was 20-77 years, with 5 cases aged below 40 years. Eight cases had long term infection and only 1 had recent infection. Two cases had fever, 1 had jaundice and none suffered from bleeding. None of the cases had travelled to Angola or Congo DR. Mosquito net use was reported by 4 cases and only 1 case reported that the house was sprayed with insecticide residual spray. None of the cases had been vaccinated against YF. Western province was experiencing an epidemic for YF virus infection. With a low prevalence, the area qualifies to be classified as a low risk for YF. Efforts to curb the epidemic are urgently needed. Yellow fever surveillance and the capacity of laboratories to diagnose YF should be strengthened.

Introduction

Yellow fever (YF) is estimated to affect about 200,000 people annually in the tropics of Africa and South America (1) and 30,000 deaths occur worldwide (2). The majority of persons infected with YF suffer from a self-limiting febrile illness. In persons who develop symptoms, symptoms occur 3-6 days after being infected and include fever, chills, severe headache, back pain, general body aches, nausea, vomiting, fatigue and weakness to severe liver disease with bleeding. Most persons who develop symptoms improve after the initial presentation of symptoms. About 15% of cases progress to a more severe form of the disease that is characterized by high fever, jaundice, bleeding, and eventually shock and failure of multiple organs (3). There is no specific treatment for yellow fever; care is based on symptoms. Steps to prevent yellow fever virus infection include using insect repellent, wearing protective clothing, and getting vaccinated (3).

Transmission of YF in Africa has been maintained by a high density of sylvatic and urban vector mosquitoes (4), mainly Aedes aegypti and Aedes africanus (5). Prevention of YF depends on avoiding mosquito bites by using repellent and wearing protective (long-sleeves, long pants and socks when outdoors) clothing and persons aged 9 months or older who live in YF endemic areas or travelling to such areas may be vaccinated to prevent infection (3).

In Africa, Yellow fever was mainly a problem of the sub-Saharan countries of West Africa, but reached as far east as central Sudan and East Africa (6-10). By 2005, Yellow fever was endemic in Angola that borders Western province of the Zambia (4). Zambia as a whole country was classified as a no risk area but Western and North-western provinces of Zambia were classified as low risk areas for yellow fever. The history behind the current classification of Western province as a low risk area for yellow fever is such that before 2005, it was classified as endemic area and in the period 2005-2010 it was removed from the list of areas with risk of transmission of yellow fever virus. The decision to classify Western province as a low potential for yellow fever exposure (11) was based on a suspected case of yellow fever that was described in North-western province of Zambia in 1943 (12), 18% seroprevalence of neutralizing antibodies to Yellow fever (13) and neighbouring areas in Angola and Democratic Republic of the Congo being at risk of yellow fever risk (11). There was no recent evidence that could have been used to classify the area. Thus, a yellow fever risk assessment survey was conducted in 2013 to provide evidence for or against the classification of the area as low risk area for yellow fever.

OUR STUDY

Western province borders with Angola and had seven districts divided into 1902 Standard Enumeration Aras (SEAs). The population stood at 881,524 with a population density of 7.0 (14). Crop and livestock production as well as fishing were the main economic activities.

Study population, sample size and sampling

This assessment was carried out among individuals aged nine months or older. The sample size calculation was based on the assumption that the seroprevalence for yellow fever was 7% based on the study conducted by Robinson (12). In estimating the sample size for persons aged 5 years or older, the following parameters were considered: a prevalence of 7%, desired precision or confidence interval (d) of $\pm$3%, and a design effect (DE) of 2 and an 80% response rate. Considering sex, we aimed to recruit 700 male and 700 female participants in each province. Assuming an average of 4 persons aged 5 years or older in each household, a total of 12 households in each of the 30 cluster were to be recruited in the survey. The total number of persons that would be recruited from each province was 1806, totalling 3612 from both provinces.

The seroprevalence of children was about half that for older children, and in estimating the sample size for persons aged below 5 years, the following parameters were considered: a prevalence of 3.5%, desired precision or confidence interval (d) of ±3.4%, and a design effect (DE) of 2 and an 80% response rate. The computed sample size was 282. Therefore, in each province 406 children would be recruited for the survey.

The sample was drawn using a two-stage cluster sampling technique using probability proportional to size. A list of the standard enumeration areas (SEAs) in each province constituted the sampling frame. The line lists of the SEAs were provided by the Government's Central Statistics Office (CSO). The sampling was designed to achieve fairly good estimates at the provincial level of analysis, and not representing the subdivisions of the province.

Data management and analysis

Data were entered in an Epi-Info data entry screen that had consistency and range checks embedded in it. Further editing was conducted by running frequencies during the analysis stage. Epi data files were exported to SPSS for data analysis. The chi-square test was used to determine associations between qualitative factors. The cut off point for statistical significance was set at the 5% level.

Ethical considerations

Ethical clearance was sought from the Tropical Diseases Research Centre Research Ethics Committee, and ethical standards were adhered to throughout this study. Informed consent was sought from study participants. Guardians provided assent for the participation of the persons under the consenting age. They were asked to read or have read to them, understand and sign/thumbprint an informed consent form. Responsible adults in the household were identified to give proxy consent on behalf of minors.

Our Findings

Altogether, 1824 persons participated in the survey of which 44.8% were males. Significantly more males (34.3%) than females (27.1%) had achieved secondary or higher levels of education ($p=0.001$). Overall, 9 (0.5%) of the participants had YF. These results are shown in Table 1.

Table 1. Description for participants in a 2013 yellow fever risk assessment in Western province

Factor	Total n (%)	Male n (%)	Female n (%)	p value
Age (years)				
<45	1503 (82.5)	679 (83.3)	823 (81.9)	0.464
45+	318 (17.5)	136 (16.7)	182 (18.1)	
Sex				
Male	815 (44.8)			
Female	1005 (55.2)			
Education				
None or primary	1256 (69.7)	528 (65.7)	727 (72.9)	0.001
Secondary or higher	546 (30.3)	276 (34.3)	270 (27.1)	
Yellow fever				
Yes	9 (0.5)	6 (0.7)	3 (0.3)	0.314
No	1815 (99.5)	809 (99.3)	1002 (99.7)	

Of the nine cases of YF, six were males. The age range of the cases was 20-77 years, with five cases aged below 40 years. Three cases had attained up to primary level of education, three had not attended school, three attained primary level of education and another three had secondary level of education.

Eight cases had long term infection and only one had recent infection. Two cases had fever, one had jaundice and none suffered from bleeding. None of the cases had travelled to Angola or Congo DR. Mosquito net use was reported by four cases and only one case reported that the house was sprayed with insecticide residual spray. Seven cases had houses with roofs made of grass and two cases house with roofs made of iron sheets. Of the nine cases, two cases had walls of houses made of mud, three had walls of houses made of poles, one had walls made of plastered cement, two had walls made of cement bricks but not plastered, and one had walls made of unburnt bricks. None of the cases had been vaccinated against YF.

DISCUSSION

This study was conducted about 50 years after the last survey on Yellow fever risk assessment was conducted. It was prompted by a reclassification of the area from a no risk to low risk area for Yellow fever. Nine cases of YF (0.5%) were identified of which eight were of long term infection and 1 was a recent infection. None of the cases had been vaccinated against YF.

The yellow fever virus was currently circulating. The prevalence of the infection in the current study is less than the 7% (12) that was reported 50 years ago in the present Western and North-western provinces. The difference in the prevalence could partly be due to differences in the stages of the epidemic. It might be that Western province was in the early stage of the epidemic, while 50 years ago when that study was conducted the area was at an advanced stage of the epidemic. Another possibility for the difference could be that North-western province that is not part of the current study could have had a higher proportion of the 7% prevalence.

All the cases of YF in the current study were adults, indicating that younger participants were less likely to have yellow fever than older participants. This finding accords that of Geser et al. (15) that the prevalence of yellow fever was positively associated with age. The increasing age with increasing seroprevalence suggests more stable rates of ongoing transmission in the population (16).

One of the reasons that were used to classify Western province as an area of low risk for yellow fever transmission was because it bordered with areas designated as having yellow fever in neighbouring Angola and DR Congo (11). Apart from North-western province that was surveyed recently, it is important that other provinces of the country be surveyed, especially Northern province that shares a border with Tanzania that has low potential for yellow fever transmission and DR Congo with most areas regarded as endemic. Resources allowing, a national survey should be conducted to clearly state the status of the country with regard to yellow fever classification.

In conclusion, Western province was experiencing an epidemic for YF virus infection. With a low prevalence, the area qualifies to be classified as a low risk for YF. Efforts to curb the epidemic are urgently needed. Yellow fever surveillance and the capacity of laboratories to diagnose YF should be strengthened.

ACKNOWLEDGMENTS

We are grateful to the interviewers for their dedicated work to successfully complete the survey. The survey could not have been successful without the cooperation of the participants and the virology laboratory staff both in Lusaka, Zambia and Dakar, Senegal for in testing samples. The survey was funded by the Ministry of Health [Zambia] and the World Health Organization.

REFERENCES

[1] Vainio J, Cutts F. Yellow Fever. Geneva: WHO Division of Emerging and other Communicable Diseases Surveilance and Control, 1998.
[2] WHO. Yellow fever. Fact sheet No100. Accessed 2014 August 08. URL:http://www.who.int/mediacentre/factsheets/fs100/en/. May 2013.
[3] Centers for Disease Control and Prevention. Yellow fever. Accessed 2014 August 08. URL:http://www.cdc.gov/yellowfever/.
[4] Barnett ED. Yellow fever: epidemiology and prevention. Clin Infect Dis 2007;44:850-6.
[5] Diallo M, Tall A, Dial I, Ba Y, Sarr FD, Ly AB, et al. Yellow feveroOutbreak in central part of Senegal 2002: Epidemiological Findings. J Public Health Epidemiol 2013;5:291-6.
[6] WHO. Yellow fever, Sudan — update. Wkly Epidemiol Rec 2012;87:477-92.
[7] Okello GBA, Agata N, Ouma J, Cherogony SC, Tukei PM, Ochieng W, den Boer JW, Sanders EJ. Outbreak of yellow fever in Kenya. Lancet 1993;341(8843):489.
[8] Haddow AJ. Yellow fever in central Uganda, 1964. I. Historical introduction. Trans R Soc Trop Med Hyg 1965;59:436–40.
[9] Reiter P, Cordellier R, Ouma JO, Cropp CB, Savage HM, Sanders EJ, et al. First recorded outbreak of yellow fever in Kenya, 1992–1993. II. Entomologic investigations. Am J Trop Med Hyg 1998;59:650–6.
[10] Bell H. Frontiers of medicine in the Anglo-Egyptian Sudan, 1899–1940. Oxford Historical Monographs. Oxford; Oxford University Press, 1999.
[11] Jentes ES, Poumerol G, Gershman MD, Hill DR, Lemarchand J, Lewis RF, et al. The revised global yellow fever risk map and recommendations for vaccination, 2010: consensus of the Informal WHO Working Group on Geographic Risk for Yellow Fever. Lancet Infect Dis 2011;11:622-32.
[12] Robinson GG. A note on mosquitoes and yellow fever in Northern Rhodesia. East Afr Med J 1950;27:284-8.
[13] Bonnel PH, Deutschman Z. Yellow fever in Africa during recent years. Bull World Health Organ 1954;11:325-89.
[14] Central Statistical Office. 2010 census of population and housing. National analytical report. Lusaka, Zambia: CSO, 2012.

[15] Geser A, Henderson BE, Christensen S. A Multipurpose Serological Survey in Kenya : 2. Results of Arbovirus Serological Tests. Bull World Health Organ 1970;43:539-52.

[16] Mease LE, Coldren RL, Musila LA, Prosser T, Ogolla F, Ofula VO, et al. Seroprevalence and distribution of arboviral infections among rural Kenyan adults: A cross-sectional study. Virology J 2011;8:371.

In: Arbovirus
Editors: S. Siziya, M. L. Mazaba et al.
ISBN: 978-1-63463-601-8

Chapter 9

DENGUE FEVER

Mazyanga L Mazaba, BSc, MSc[1*],
Olusegun Babaniyi, MBBS, MPH, MSc[1],
Mwaka Monza, MBChB, PhD[2],
Idah Mweene-Ndumba, BSc, MPH[1],
David Mulenga, BSc, MPH[3],
Freddie Masaninga, BSc, MSc, PhD[1],
Peter Songolo, MBChB, MPH[1],
Francis Kasolo, MBChB, MPH[4],
and Seter Siziya, BA(Ed), MSc, PhD[5,6]

[1]World Health Organization, Lusaka, Zambia
[2]University Teaching Hospital, Lusaka, Zamia
[3]School of Medicine, Copperbelt University, Ndola, Zambia
[4]World Health Organization, AFRO region, Congo Brazzaville
[5]School of Medicine, Copperbelt University, Ndola, Zambia
[6]University of Lusaka, Lusaka, Zambia

Dengue virus infection has become a major public health concern worldwide, although it has not been reported before in Zambia. The objective of the study was to determine the prevalence and correlates for

* Correspondence: Mazyanga L Mazaba, EPI Unit, World Health Organization, Lusaka, Zambia and Virology Unit, University Teaching Hospital, Lusaka, Zambia. E-mail: mazmazli@yahoo.com.

dengue virus infection in Western province of Zambia. Secondary data, obtained in a yellow fever risk assessment survey, was used in the study. A total of 1,823 persons were investigated of whom 55.2% were female and 25.1% were in the 5-14 years age group. Overall, 7.1% (7.2% males and 7.0% females; p=0.887) were infected with dengue virus. Persons in the age group 25-34 years were 66% (AOR=1.66; 95% CI [1.09, 2.54]) more likely to have the infection compared to those aged 45 years or older. Persons who had attained primary education were 37% (AOR= 1.37; 95% CI [(1.05, 1.78]) more likely to have the infection than those who had higher levels of education. Persons who had travelled to Angola were 2.11 times (AOR= 2.11; 95% CI [1.41, 3.15]) more likely to have the infection compared to those who had not travelled to Angola. Surveillance should be strengthened at the border in order to curtail the epidemic.

INTRODUCTION

Dengue is a mosquito-borne (Aedes aegypti) systemic viral infection found in tropical and sub-tropical regions and has become a major public health concern worldwide (1). The complications of dengue infection (Dengue Haemorrhagic Fever or Dengue Shock Syndrome) are life-threatening in those with chronic diseases and asthma (2). Major epidemics caused by dengue fever occurred from the 17th to early 20th centuries (3). It is estimated that close to 4 billion persons living in 128 countries are at risk of dengue infection (4), with the virus being endemic in over 110 countries. The endemic countries are in Africa, the Americas, the Eastern Mediterranean, South-east Asia and Western Pacific. Severely affected regions including the Americas, the Eastern Mediterranean, South-east Asia and Western Pacific reported more than 1.2 million and 2.3 million cases in 2008 and 2010 respectively.

Dengue epidemics in Africa have increased since 1980 with most activity documented in East Africa (5). Most recently outbreaks have been reported in Angola (6), and Kenya (7). Dengue is now one of most important tropical diseases second to malaria causing approximately 50 to 100 million cases of DF and 500,000 cases of DHF (8). The public health impact of dengue is greatly underestimated because of poor surveillance data (9). Though the factors responsible for the dramatic resurgence of epidemic dengue are not fully understood, it appears it is closely associated with demographic and societal changes over the past 50 years (10).

The relationship between age and risk of dengue fever has not been consistent. According to Egger and Coleman (11), the risk for age in relation to classic dengue fever had never been quantified. Using data from clinical patients, Egger and Coleman showed that the risk of classical dengue after primary dengue increases with age. Another study revealed that classic dengue is primarily common among older children and adults (12,13). The epidemiologic characteristics of dengue differ by region and the incidence by age (14-16). A study by Anker and Amina indicated a consistent pattern of male predominance in the reported number of dengue cases among 15 years or older in six Asian countries (17). Travel (18) and education (19) have also been documented to be associated with Dengue fever.

Zambia recently (in 2013) carried out a yellow fever risk assessment in Western and North-Western provinces. Positive cases for dengue fever were identified amongst the study population in the survey. This paper documents the prevalence and correlated for dengue fever in Western province.

OUR STUDY

Western province borders with Angola and had seven districts divided into 1,902 Standard Enumeration Areas (SEAs). The population stood at 881,524 with a population density of 7.0. Crop and livestock production as well as fishing were the main economic activities (20).

Study population, Sample size, inclusion/exclusion criteria and sampling

The survey was carried out among individuals aged nine months or older. The sample size calculation was based on the assumption that the seroprevalence for yellow fever was 7% based on the study on yellow fever conducted by Robinson (21). For persons aged 5 years or older, the following parameters were considered in estimating the sample size, a prevalence of 7%, desired precision or confidence interval (d) of $\pm$3%, and a design effect (DE) of 2 and an 80% response rate. The study aimed to recruit 700 male and 700 female participants in each province. A total of 12 households in each of the 30 clusters, assuming an average of 4 persons aged 5 years or older in each household, were to be recruited in the survey. The total number of persons that would be recruited from each province was 1806, totalling 3612 from both provinces.

The seroprevalence of children below the age of five years was about half that for older persons, and in estimating the sample size for persons aged below 5 years, the following parameters were considered: a prevalence of 3.5%, desired precision or confidence interval (d) of ±3.4%, and a design effect (DE) of 2 and an 80% response rate. The computed sample size was 282. A total of 406 children would be recruited in each province for the survey.

Any individual aged 9 months or older and who was a member of a sampled household and resident in the study site for at least seven days was requested to participate in the survey. Individuals who received yellow fever vaccination in the last ten years were eligible to participate in the survey. Exclusion criteria left out any person, who was either less than 9 months of age or any person, regardless of age, who resided in the study site for a period of less than seven days prior to the survey. Children under the age of nine months raises the risk of false positive results as children under this age may still carry maternal antibodies from immunized or exposed mothers.

A two-stage cluster sampling technique using probability proportional to size was used to draw the sample. A list of the standard enumeration areas (SEAs) in each province constituted the sampling frame. The sampling was designed to achieve fairly good estimates at the provincial level of analysis, and not representing the subdivisions of the province.

Study variables

Dependent variable

A case with evidence of dengue infection exposure was defined as any individual aged 9 months or older whose blood sample was confirmed to have dengue virus exposure through the detection of dengue virus-specific IgG and IgM antibodies.

Independent variables

The independent variables included age, sex, occupation, history of travel to Angola and/or DRC and use of mosquito preventive measures.

Laboratory procedure

About 3 to 5 millilitres of blood was collected by venepuncture into an EDTA vacutainer tube and transported on cold chain to the local laboratories for serum separation and storage. Samples were subjected to primary testing (yellow fever virus specific IgG and IgM) at the University of Teaching Hospital in Zambia virology unit and Institute Pasteur, Dakar. All presumptive yellow fever virus specific IgG and IgM samples were subjected to IgG and IgM antibodies against other flaviviruses known to cause haemorrhagic fever-like disease including dengue.

Data management and analysis

Data were entered in an Epi-Info data entry screen that had consistency and range checks embedded in it. Further editing was conducted by running frequencies during the analysis stage. Epi data files were exported to SPSS for data analysis. The data was summarized to describe the occurrence of dengue virus exposed individuals in absolute numbers and percentage by place (residence, travel or work) and person (age, sex, occupation). Further analysis was conducted to determine independent factors associated with yellow fever seropositivity. Odds ratios were used to estimate magnitudes of associations.

Ethical considerations

Ethical clearance was sought from the Tropical Diseases Research Centre Research Ethics Committee, and ethical standards were adhered to throughout this study. Informed consent was sought from study participants. Guardians provided assent for the participation of the persons under the consenting age. Participants were asked to read or have read to them, understand and sign/thumbprint an informed consent form. Responsible adults in the household were identified to give proxy consent on behalf of minors.

OUR FINDINGS

A total of 1,823 persons were investigated (questionnaires and laboratory tests) for dengue virus in Western province. Overall, 55.2% of the participants were female and 25.1% were in the age group 5-14 years. Altogether, 48.2% of all persons sampled had attained primary education. Males tended to be more educated than females (p=0.002). No significant association was observed between sex and dengue virus infection. Overall, 7.1% of the participants in western province had previous dengue. These results are shown in table 1.

Table 1. Sample description for Western province for dengue virus infection

Factor	Total n (%)	Male n (%)	Female n (%)	p value
Age (years)				
<5	184 (10.1)	81 (9.9)	102 (10.1)	0.131
5-14	471 (25.1)	231 (28.3)	240 (23.9)	
15-24	390 (21.4)	180 (22.1)	210 (20.9)	
25-34	245 (13.5)	94 (11.5)	151 (15.0)	
35-44	213 (11.7)	93 (11.4)	120 (11.9)	
45+	318 (17.5)	136 (16.7)	182 (18.1)	
Sex				
Male	815 (44.8)	-	-	-
Female	1005 (55.2)	-	-	
Education				
None	388 (21.5)	152 (18.9)	235 (23.6)	0.002
Primary	868 (48.2)	376 (46.8)	492 (49.3)	
Secondary or higher	546 (30.3)	276 (34.3)	270 (27.1)	
Dengue virus infection				
Yes	130 (7.1)	59 (7.2)	70 (7.0)	0.887
No	1693 (92.9)	755 (92.8)	935 (93.0)	

* Numbers may not add up due to missing information.

Of the factors considered in bivariate analysis age, education, and visit to Angola were significantly associated with risk of dengue infection (see table 2). After adjusting for other factors in multivariate analysis, those in the age group 25-34 years were 66% (AOR=1.66; 95% CI [1.09, 2.54]) more likely to have dengue infection compared to those aged 45 years or older. Those who had attained primary education were 37% (AOR= 1.37; 95% CI [(1.05, 1.78]) more likely to have dengue infection than those who had attained secondary education or higher. In relation to visitation to Angola, those who visited were 2.11 times (AOR= 2.11; 95% CI [1.41, 3.15]) more likely to have dengue infection.

Table 2. Factors associated with dengue virus infection in logistic regression analysis for Western province

Factor	OR (95% CI)	AOR (95% CI)
Age (years)		
<5	0.43 (0.20, 0.91)	0.54 (0.24, 1.24)
5-14	0.71 (0.47, 1.08)	0.63 (0.40, 0.98)
15-24	0.96 (0.63, 1.44)	1.02 (0.66, 1.58)
25-34	1.66 (1.10, 2.50)	1.66 (1.09, 2.54)
35-44	0.83 (0.48, 1.43)	0.76 (0.44, 1.32)
45+	1	1
Sex		
Male	1.02 (0.85, 1.22)	-
Female	1	
Education		
None	0.84 (0.61, 1.16)	0.89 (0.62, 1.29)
Primary	1.31 (1.03, 1.67)	1.37 (1.05, 1.78)
Secondary or higher	1	1
Use of mosquito net		
Yes	1.13 (0.94, 1.36)	-
No	1	
Insecticide Residual Spraying		
Yes	1.14 (0.90, 1.44)	-
No	1	
Visited Congo DRC		
Yes	1.62 (0.55,4.75)	-
No	1	
Visited Angola		
Yes	2.41 (1.65, 3.52)	2.11 (1.41, 3.15)
No	1	1

DISCUSSION

There is no documentation of a previous survey except for a confirmed case of a European traveller/expatriate who was in Zambia between 1987 and 1993 (22). This study reveals a prevalence of dengue infection in Western province at 7.1% with those in the age group 25-34 being more likely to be affected. Respondents with lower than secondary school qualification, as well as those who travelled to Angola were more likely to be associated with dengue infection.

The factors responsible for epidemic dengue as a global public health problem in the past 17 years are complex and not fully understood. However, demographic changes over the past 50 years have been associated with dengue (12). There are inconsistencies in the description of the relationship between age and risk of dengue infection. Some studies cite the younger age as more likely to get dengue infection, others cite increasing infection rate with increasing age (23). Epidemiological data on dengue infection in Brazil indicates changing age group patterns (24).

Travel has been documented to be associated with increase in the spread of Dengue virus from endemic to non-endemic areas. The continued spread of dengue has been supported by global trade and increasing travel within and between countries (25). Travel whether by air, motor vehicles or foot, increases the risk of introducing arthropod-borne virus diseases including dengue fever from endemic to non-endemic areas (23). With small scale cross border trading, want for closer health facilities, and family ties across borders, there is increasing travel between the dengue endemic neighbouring country of Angola and Zambia. Angola is currently having a dengue epidemic (26) and this could have facilitated the introduction of dengue virus and infection in Zambia.

The finding in the current study that education was related to infection was not consistent (no gradient in the odds of being infected among the levels of education) in that while persons who had no formal education were equally likely to have the infection as those who had secondary or higher levels of education, persons who had primary level of education were more likely to have infection compared to those who had higher levels of education. Results from a study in urban areas in Thailand indicated that persons who earned secondary or higher levels of education had a higher risk for being infected than those who earned elementary or lower levels of education (19). Contrary to the explanation of such phenomena by Koyadun et al. (19) that persons who have a high level of schooling may have a higher chance to get skilled careers and seek jobs far away from their community where they would increase their risk of getting infection, it is not clear what factors would put both persons with no formal education and persons with secondary or higher levels of education at equal chances of getting the infection. Further studies are needed to elucidate the relationship between education and dengue virus infection. In order to curtail the epidemic in Western province of Zambia, surveillance at border posts should be enhanced through screening of persons crossing the border and strengthening laboratory capacity to detect infection.

ACKNOWLEDGMENTS

The survey could not have been successful without the cooperation of the participants. We acknowledge the laboratory support received from Virology laboratory staff, University Teaching Hospital, Lusaka, Zambia and Institute de Pasteur, Dakar, Senegal. We are grateful to the interviewers for their dedicated work to successfully complete the survey. The survey was funded by the Ministry of Health [Zambia] and the World Health Organization.

REFERENCES

[1] Centers for Disease Control and Prevention. Dengue. Accessed 2010 August 31. URL: www.cdc.gov/dengue/.

[2] Guzman MG, Halstead SB, Artsob H, Buchy P, Farrar J, Gubler DJ, et al. Dengue: a continuing global threat. Nat Rev Microbiol 2010;8(Suppl 12) S7–16.

[3] Gubler DJ. Dengue and dengue hemorrhagic fever: its history and resurgence as a global public health problem. In: Gubler DJ, Kuno G, eds. Dengue and dengue hemorrhagic fever. London: CAB International, 1997:1-22.

[4] Brady OJ, Gething PW, Bhatt S. Refining the global spatial limits of dengue virus transmission by evidence-based consensus. Nature 2013;496(7446):504-7.

[5] Gubler DJ. Dengue. In: Monath TPM, ed. Epidemiology of arthropodborne viral disease, Boca Raton (FL): CRC Press, 1988:223-60.

[6] Centers for Disease Control and Prevention. Ongoing dengue epidemic - Angola, June 2013. MMWR 2013;62:504-7.

[7] Mease LE, Coldren RL, Musila LA, Prosser T, Ogolla F, Ofula VO, et al. Seroprevalence and distribution of arboviral infections among rural Kenyan adults: a cross-sectional study. Virology J 2011;8:371.

[8] World Health Organization. Global alert and response. Impact of dengue. Accessed 2014 August 31. URL: http://www.who.int/csr/disease/dengue/impact/en/index.htm

[9] Gubler DJ. Resurgent vector-borne diseases as a global health problem. Emerg Infect Dis 1998;4:442-50.

[10] Gubler D. The emergence of epidemic dengue fever and dengue hemorrhagic fever in the Americas: a case of failed public health policy. Rev Panam Salud Publica 2005;17:221-4.

[11] Egger JR, Coleman PG. Age and clinical dengue illness. Emerg Infect Dis 2007;13:924-7.

[12] Gubler DJ. Dengue and dengue hemorrhagic fever. Clin Microbiol Rev 1998;11:480-96.

[13] Hayes EB, Gubler DJ. Dengue and dengue hemorrhagic fever. Pediatr Infect Dis J. 1992;11:311-7.

[14] Cavalcanti LP, Vilar D, Souza-Santos R, Teixeira MG. Change in age pattern of persons with dengue, northeastern Brazil. Emerg Infect Dis 2011;17(1):132-4.

[15] Halstead SB. Dengue in the Americas and Southeast Asia: do they differ? Rev Panam Salud Publica 2006;20:407-15.

[16] Teixeira MG, Costa Mda C, Barreto F, Barreto ML. Dengue: twenty-five years since reemergence in Brazil. Cad Saude Publica 2009;25 Suppl 1:S7-18.

[17] Anker M, Arima Y. Male-female differences in the number of reported incident dengue fever cases in six Asian countries. Western Pac Surveill Response J 2011;2:17-23.

[18] Blackburn NK, Rawat R. Dengue fever imported from India. A report of 3 cases. S Afr Med. 1987;71:386-7.

[19] Koyadun S, Butraporn P, Kittayapong P. Ecologic and sociodemographic risk determinants for dengue transmission in urban areas in Thailand. Interdiscip Perspect Infect Dis 2012, Article ID 907494, 12 pages. doi:10.1155/2012/907494.

[20] Central Statistical Office (CSO), Ministry of Health (MOH), Tropical Diseases Research Centre (TDRC), University of Zambia, and Macro International Inc. Zambia Demographic and Health Survey 2007. Calverton, MD: CSO Macro International, 2009.

[21] Robinson GG. A note on mosquitoes and yellow fever in Northern Rhodesia. East Afr Med J 1950;27:284-8.

[22] Amarasinghe A, Kuritsk JN, Letson GW, Margolis HS. Dengue virus infection in Africa. Emerg Infect Dis 2011;17:1349-54.

[23] Blackburn NK, Rawat R. Dengue fever imported from India: a report of 3 cases. S Afr Med J 1987;71:386-7.

[24] Cavalcanti LP, Vilar D, Souza-Santos R, Teixeira MG. Change in age pattern of persons with dengue, northeastern Brazil. Emerg Infect Dis 2011;17:132-4)

[25] Cameron P. Simmons CP, Farrar JJ, van Vinh Chau N, Wills B. Dengue. N Engl J Med 2012;366:1423-32.

[26] Centers for Disease Control and Prevention. Dengue in Angola. Accessed 2013 May 24. URL: http://wwwnc.cdc.gov/travel/notices/watch/dengue-angola.

In: Arbovirus
Editors: S. Siziya, M. L. Mazaba et al.
ISBN: 978-1-63463-601-8

Chapter 10

DISTRIBUTION OF ZIKA VIRUS INFECTION SPECIFIC IGG IN WESTERN PROVINCE OF ZAMBIA

Olusegun Babaniyi[1], Peter Songolo[1,*], Mazyanga L Mazaba[1], Idah Mweene-Ndumba[1], Freddie Masaninga[1], Emmanuel Rudatsikira[2] and Seter Siziya[3,4]

[1]World Health Organization, Lusaka, Zambia
[2]School of Health Professionals, Andrews University, Michigan, United States of America
[3]School of Medicine, Copperbelt University, Ndola, Zambia
[4]University of Lusaka, Lusaka, Zambia

Zika virus (ZIKV) is a flavivirus that causes disease with similar but milder symptoms to dengue fever. There is no information on Zika virus infection in Zambia. Hence, the objective was to study was to determine the prevalence and correlates for Zika virus infection in Western province of Zambia. A cross-sectional study using a standardised questionnaire was conducted. Logistic regression analyses were conducted to determine factors associated with Zika virus infection. Out of 1824 respondents, 44.8% were males and 36.0% were aged below 15 years. Altogether, 10.2% of the participants had Zika virus infection. Factors associated

* Corresponding author: Peter Songolo, MBChB, MPH, World Health Organization, Lusaka, Zambia. E-mail: songolop@who.int.

with the infection were age and education. Participants aged less than 15 years were 53% (AOR=0.47, 95% CI [0.34, 0.65]) less likely to be infected compared to those aged 45 years or older. Compared to participants who had attained secondary or higher levels of education, those who had attained primary level of education were 1.28 (95% CI [1.04, 1.58]) times more likely to have the infection. Zika virus infection is prevalent among the residents of Western Province in Zambia. There is need to strengthen strategies to address the emerging challenge of Zika virus infection such as laboratory diagnostic capacities.

INTRODUCTION

Zika virus (ZIKV) is a flavivirus that causes disease with similar but milder symptoms to dengue fever. Clinical pictures range from asymptomatic cases to an influenza-like syndrome associated to fever, headache, malaise and cutaneous rash (1). Other less frequent symptoms and signs of ZIKV include myalgia, headache, retro-orbital pain, oedema and vomiting (2). Its natural transmission cycle in Africa involves primarily mosquitoes (*Aedes* species) and monkeys. While serological and entomological Zika virus infection have been reported in different areas in Africa including Burkina Faso, Ivory Coast, Egypt, Central African Republic, Mozambique, Nigeria, Uganda and Senegal, entomological and virological surveillance for arboviruses have been conducted since 1972 in Senegal and revealed presence of Zika virus (3). The virus was first identified in 1947 in rhesus monkey serum from Zika forest in Uganda (4). However ZIKV antibodies have been detected in humans across Africa, and Asia (5,6). In Cameroon, the infection with Zika virus spread to neighbouring Nigeria resulting in an epidemic with symptoms including jaundice (7), an indicator for potential for global spread (8).

Despite the widespread distribution of Zika virus, there have been very few reported human cases until the Yap outbreak in 2007 (9). In particular, there is no documented information on Zika virus infection in Western province of Zambia. Following a risk assessment for Yellow fever in Western province of Zambia resulting from a re-classification of the province by World Health Organization as a low-risk area for Yellow fever, a study was undertaken using data collected from the Yellow fever survey to determine the prevalence and correlates for Zika virus infection in Western province of Zambia.

Our study

Western Province has a common border with Angola. The geography of the province is dominated by the Barotse Floodplain of the Zambezi river. This floodplain is inundated from December to June; this is important to agriculture as it provides natural irrigation for the grasslands. Much of the province is covered by sand believed to come from the Kalahari Desert, grasslands and woodlands.

Western Province had seven districts with a total of 1,902 Standard Enumeration Aras (SEAs). Fishing and cattle rearing were the main occupation in the province. The population of the province was 854,890 according to national census of 2010 (10).

Western province borders with Angola and had seven districts divided into 1,902 SEAs. The population stood at 881,524 with a population density of 7.0 (10). Crop and livestock production as well as fishing were the main economic activities.

Sample sizes

The sample size calculation was based on the assumption that the sero-prevalence for Yellow fever was 7% based on the study conducted by Robinson (11). A Statcal program in Epi Info v6.04 was used to estimate the sample size. The sample size was equally allocated to North-Western and Western provinces and powered to avoid chance findings, that is, 1,800 participants from each province.

Sampling

A multi-stage sampling technique was used for participants in both districts. Firstly, wards were randomly selected from each constituency. In the second stage of sampling, standard enumeration areas (SEAs) proportional to the ward size were systematically sampled. All survey participants aged nine months or older in a selected household were eligible to be enrolled in the study.

Ethical approval

The study protocol was reviewed and approved by the Tropical Diseases Research Centre Research Ethics Committee, and permission to conduct the study was obtained from the Ministry of Health, Zambia. Informed consent was obtained from survey participants after the interviewer had explained the benefits and risks of participating in the study. Entry forms were viewed only by those approved to be part of the survey.

Data collection

A detailed semi structured questionnaire was used to collect information. The questionnaires were pre-tested to validate the appropriateness of the questions to capture the required information. During the data collection process, questionnaires were checked for inconsistencies and completeness on a daily basis.

Data management and analysis

All data were entered into a computer using an Epi-Info data entry screen that had consistency and range checks embedded in it. The Epi data file was exported to SPSS for data analysis. Further editing was conducted by running frequencies during the analysis stage. Odds ratios were used to estimate magnitudes of associations using unadjusted odds ratios (OR) and adjusted odds ratios (AOR) together with their 95% confidence intervals (CI).

OUR FINDINGS

A total of 1,824 participants out of which 44.8% were males participated in the survey. The age distribution was similar between sexes with 36.0% of the participants belonging to the under 15 years age group. A significant association between education and sex was observed ($p=0.002$) with 34.3% of males and 27.1% of females having attained secondary or higher levels of education

Table 1. Sample description for Western province for Zika virus infection

Factor	Total n (%)	Male n (%)	Female n (%)	p value
Age (years)				
< 15	655 (36.0)	312 (38.3)	342 (34.0)	0.122
15 – 24	390 (21.4)	180 (22.1)	210 (20.9)	
25 – 34	245 (13.5)	94 (11.5)	151 (15.0)	
35 – 44	213 (11.5)	93 (11.4)	120 (11.9)	
45+	318 (17.5)	136 (16.7)	182 (18.1)	
Sex				
Male	815 (44.8)			
Female	1005 (55.2)			
Education				
None	388 (21.5)	152 (18.9)	235 (23.6)	0.002
Primary	868 (48.2)	376 (46.8)	492 (49.3)	
Secondary or higher	546 (30.3)	276 (34.3)	270 (27.1)	
Zika virus infection				
Yes	186 (10.2)	82 (10.1)	103 (10.2)	0.957
No	1638 (89.8)	733 (89.9)	902 (89.9)	

Altogether, 10.2% of the participants had Zika virus infection with no sex difference (p=0.957). Table 1 shows the description of the sample. While age, education and visiting Angola were significantly associated with Zika virus infection in bivariate analyses, only age and education remained significantly associated with the infection in multivariate analysis. Participants aged less 15 years were observed to be 53% (AOR=0.47, 95% CI [0.34, 0.65]) less likely to have the infection compared to participants of age 45 years or older. Meanwhile, participants who had attained primary level of education were 28% (AOR=1.28, 95% CI [1.04, 1.58]) more likely to have the infection compared to participants who had attained secondary or higher levels of education.

Discussion

Zika virus which had not been previously reported in Western province of Zambia was prevalent affecting 10.2% of the survey participants. Compared to other findings, the prevalence in the current study is much lower than what has been reported elsewhere in Africa. The findings in Nigeria, reporting rates of 31 and 56% (12,13) and in Yap island of Federated States of Micronesia reporting a rate of 73% (14) were based on small sample sizes, and this may partly explain the differences in the rates reported.

While age was significantly associated with Zika infection in the current study, no significant association was observed between age and the infection on the Yap island (14). However, in a study conducted in Kenya, age was significantly associated with the infection. The risk of infection linearly increased with age (15). Older persons may have been more exposed to infection than the younger ones partly due to activities such as social gathering and economic activities such as fishing, crop and livestock production that may predispose them to mosquito bites. Repellents may not be affordable in poor communities. Wearing of long sleeved shorts and trousers for men and wearing of wrappers, traditionally known as *chitenge*, by women may be possible alternatives to minimize man-mosquito contact.

The association between education and Zika virus infection was not consistent. While persons who had never been to school were equally likely to be infected as those with secondary or higher levels of education, persons who had attained primary level of education were more likely to be infected compared to persons with higher levels of education. Further analysis is needed to consider possible confounding factors such as the wealth index in the relationship between education and infection. Alternatively, persons with primary level of education may be more engaged in activities, for which we are unable to suggest, that may predispose them to mosquito carrying the infection.

Despite the fact that a high proportion of samples collected during the risk assessment tested positive for Zika virus infection (10.2%), no human case of Zika disease had been reported from Western province. This may be due to the lack of knowledge by the medical personnel and partly due to the absence of a case definition for Zika virus infection in the Integrated Diseases Surveillance and Response (IDSR) guidelines which are widely used for syndromic disease surveillance in Zambia. Furthermore, the symptoms of Zika infection apart from being sub-clinical in presentation could mimick malaria which is prevalent in the province. Therefore, suspected malaria cases may mask outbreaks of Zika virus infection. Grard et al. (16) in their study observed that the number of human cases of Zika virus infection were few compared to Dengue virus infection probably due to the occurrence of sub-clinical form of Zika disease that did not require medical attention.

Table 2. Factors associated with Zika virus infection in Western Province in bivariate and multivariate logistic regression analyses

Factor	OR (95% CI)	AOR (95% CI)
Age (years)		
< 15	0.51 (0.38, 0.69)	0.47 (0.34, 0.65)
15 – 24	0.74 (0.53, 1.02)	0.81 (0.57, 1.13)
25 – 34	1.19 (0.85, 1.67)	1.24 (0.88, 1.74)
35 – 44	1.03 (0.71, 1.50)	1.03 0.71, 1.48)
45+	1	1
Sex		
Male	0.99 (0.85, 1.15)	
Female	1	
Education		
None	0.92 (0.71, 1.19)	1.02 (0.77, 1.34)
Primary	1.23 (1.00, 1,51)	1.28 (1.04, 1,58)
Secondary or higher	1	1
Use of mosquito nets		
Yes	0.98 (0.84, 1.15)	_
No	1	
In-door Residual Spraying		
Yes	0.90 (0.72, 1.14)	_
No	1	
Visited Angola		
Yes	1.67 (1.12, 2.50)	_
No	1	

The other challenge contributing to lack of information on arboviral disease is the limitations on availability of diagnostic methods, thereby making it difficult to identify these emerging diseases in the country. Brady et al. in assessing the distribution of dengue in the entire continent alluded to this challenge in many healthcare settings coupled with scanty information or data on surveillance and research generated reports in many resource poor countries (17).

The discovery of ZIKV in the Western Province of Zambia strongly indicates the need to develop laboratory capacity for diagnosis of flaviviruses and strengthen Integrated Disease Surveillance and Response (IDSR). Strengthening the capacities of the laboratory is key to confirming clinically suspicious cases. There is need to strengthen control measures for malaria as the vector is similar and as such the country should scale-up the use of Insecticide-treated nets (ITNs) and in-door residual spraying to reduce human mosquito contact. Other measures include health education to promote personal protection using long-sleeved clothes and repellents. Furthermore, although research efforts have focused on many of these viruses, other medically important members of the mosquito-borne flaviviruses, such as Zika virus, have received far less attention.

REFERENCES

[1] Faye O, Freire CCM, Iamarino A, Faye O, de Oliveira JVC, Molecular evolution of Zika virus during its emergence in the 20th century. PLoS Negl Trop Dis 2014;8:2636.

[2] Hayes EB. Zika virus outside Africa. Emerg Infect Dis 2013;15:1347-9.

[3] Faye O, Faye O, Diallo D, Diallo M, Weidman M, Sall AA. Quantitative real-time PCR detection of Zika virus and evaluation with filed-caught mosquitoes. Virol J 2013;10:311.

[4] Whelan P, Hall J. Zika virus disease, The Northern Territory Disease Control Bulletin. 2008;15:19-21.

[5] Tappe D, Rissland J, Gabriel M, Emmerich P, Günther S, Held G, et al. First case of laboratory-confirmed Zika virus infection imported into Europe, November 2013. Euro surveill 2014;19:1-3.

[6] Faye O, Faye O, Freire CCM, de Oliviera JV, Rubing C, Zanotto PMA, et al. Molecular evolution of Zika virus, an neglected emerging disease in Africa and Asia. BMC Proc 2011;5:59.

[7] Fokam EB, Levai LD, Guzman H, Amelia PA, Titanji VPK, Tesh RB, et al. Silent circulation of arboviruses in Cameroon. East Afr Med J 2010;87:262-7.

[8] Grard G, Moureau G, Charrel RN, Holmes EC, Gould EA, de Lamballerie X; Genomics and evolution of Aedes-borne flaviviruses. J Gen Virol, 2010;91:87-94.

[9] Duffy MR, Chen T-H, Hancock WT, Powers AM, Kool JL, Lanciotti RS, et al. Zika virus outbreak on Yap island, Federated States of Micronesia. New Engl J Med 2009;360:2536-43.

[10] Central Statistical Office. 2010 census of population and housing. National analytical report. Lusaka, Zambia: CSO, 2012.

[11] Robinson GG. A note on mosquitoes and yellow fever in Northern Rhodesia. East Afr Med J 1950;27:284-8.

[12] Fagbami AH. Zika virus infections in Nigeria: virological and seroepidemiological investigations in Oyo State. J Hyg Camb 1979;83:213-9.

[13] Adekolu-John EO, Fagbami AH. Arthropod-borne virus antibodies in sera of rfesidents of Kainji lake basin, Nigeria 1980. Trans R Soc Trop Med Hyg 1983;77:149-51.

[14] Duffy MR, Chen T-H, Hancock TW, Powers AM, Kool JL, Lanciotti RS, et al. Zika virus outbreak on Yap island, Federated States of Micronesia. N Eng J Med 2009;360:2536-43.

[15] Geser A, Henderson BE, Christensen S. A multipurpose serological survey in Kenya. Bull World Health Organ 1970;43:539-52.

[16] Grard G, Caron M, Mombo IM, Nkoghe D, Ondo SM, Jiolle D, et al. Zika virus in Gabon (Central Africa) – 2007: a new threat from Aedes albopictus? PLoS Negl Trop Dis 2014;8:e2681.

[17] Brady OJ, Gething PW, Bhatt S, Messina JP, Brownstein JS, Hoen AG, et al. Refining the global spatial limits of dengue virus transmission by evidence-based consensus. PLoS Negl Trop Dis, 2012;6:e1760.

In: Arbovirus
Editors: S. Siziya, M. L. Mazaba et al.
ISBN: 978-1-63463-601-8

Chapter 11

WEST NILE VIRUS INFECTION: ASSESSING THE CONTRIBUTING FACTORS

Idah Mweene-Ndumba[1,3], Seter Siziya[2], Mwaka Monze[3], Mazyanga L Mazaba[1,3], Freddie Masaninga[1], Peter Songolo[1], Peter Mwaba[4] and Olusegun A Babaniyi[1,*]

[1]World Health Organization, Lusaka, Zambia,
[2]School of Medicine, Copperbelt University, Ndola, Zambia/ University of Lusaka, Lusaka, Zambia,
[3]University Teaching Hospital, Lusaka, Zambia,
[4]Ministry of Home Affairs, Lusaka, Zambia

West Nile virus (WNV) infection has been reported worldwide with varying prevalence rates within countries. The purpose of this study was to determine the extent of WNV infection and its correlates in Western province of Zambia. The study used secondary data that was collected in a yellow fever risk assessment survey. Logistic regression analyses were used to determine correlates for infection. A total of 1824 respondents participated in the survey of which 55.2% were females. The prevalence of WNV infection was 18.3%. Participants aged below 15 years were 61% (AOR 0.39 95% CI [0.30-0.51]) less likely to be infected with WNV compared to those above 15 years of age. Participants who attained

* Corresponding author: Idah Mweene-Ndumba, BSc, MPH, World Health Organization, Lusaka, Zambia. E-mail: idahndumba12@gmail.com.

primary level education were 44% (AOR 1.44, 95% CI [1.22-1.70]) more likely to be infected than those who attained secondary and higher levels of education. Participants who travelled to Angola were 78% (AOR, 1.78, 95% CI [1.25-2.55]) more likely to be infected with the virus than those who did not travel. WNV infection is common in Western province, and interventions should be designed taking into account the correlates for WNV infection that have been identified in the current study.

INTRODUCTION

West Nile virus (WNV), an arthropod-borne Flavivirus, is transmitted to human beings through a mosquito bite of the *culex* species (1). The life cycle of WNV is primarily between birds and mosquitoes and human beings are infected by mosquito bites when the normal cycle has been broken (1). Of those that are infected by the virus 1:4 become ill and less than 1% develop severe symptoms (nueroinvasive disease) such as meningitis, encephalitis and acute flaccid paralysis. WNV infection has a case fatality rate of 10% among the severe cases (1,2,5). Most of the infections are usually asymptomatic but those who show symptoms come down with headaches, myalgia, arthralgia and rash (6). Currently no treatment exists for arboviral diseases and there are no licensed vaccines for humans, therefore preventive measures against infection with WNV are encouraged (1,4).

WNV human infections have been reported worldwide after being first discovered in Uganda in 1937 (5,6) with reports in Africa, Asia, Australia, Europe and the United States of America (7). The seroprevalence studies in these countries have shown prevalence rate variations within countries with some parts of the country having higher rates than the other (8). At present up to 30,584 cases and 1,214 deaths have been reported to CDC, which is a major health threat and assessment of the factors leading to the disease was needed (2). In America, strategies to identify the risk factors to human infections had been put in place (2). Risk factors for WNV infection are not properly defined except the common ones such as mosquito control measures, avoiding exposure to mosquito bites and use of insect repellent which have been reported to have proved to have reduced the disease (1,4).

Several risk factors for WNV infection such as climate and environmental factors emerged from studies in America. High population density was significantly associated with the viral transmission even after adjusting for other environmental factors (2) and the results were comparable to results obtained in other studies which confirmed an association between urban/sub-urban versus a more rural area (9,10). However other studies reported significant association when there was less population density and rural. Temperature changes determining human activity and mosquito replication was also significantly associated with risk of infection. It was also concluded that these factors could differ yearly due to changes in bird populations with high bird population as being protective (2). It is possible that when there are more birds the virus could be concentrated in bird-mosquito-bird cycle whereas if there are fewer birds the mosquito could resort to human meals. Studies have also confirmed that age has a bearing on the severity of the infection with the older age group, 50 years or older, being most at risk (2). In Arizona, staying at home and not attending school were found to be risk factors for WNV infection, although it was argued that the possibility that those who stayed at home were the elderly who were already known to be at high risk of infection with WNV (1).

There is knowledge gap concerning WNV infections in Zambia and particularly in Western province despite the province being neighbors with countries which are endemic with the disease. The purpose of this analysis was to determine the extent of WNV infection and to assess its correlates in Western province of Zambia.

OUR STUDY

The study was conducted in Western province of Zambia. The selection of the province was based on its re-classification as low potential risk area for yellow fever transmission by World Health Organization in 2010 (11). Western province with a population of 881,524 (12), borders with Angola and has seven districts divided into 1,902 Standard Enumeration Areas (SEAs). The main economic activities were crop farming, livestock production and fishing.

Study population, Sample size, inclusion/exclusion criteria and sampling

This assessment was carried out among individuals aged nine months or older. In estimating the sample size for persons aged 5 years or older, the following parameters were considered: a prevalence of 7%, desired precision or confidence interval (d) of ±3%, and a design effect (DE) of 2 and an 80%

response rate. Considering sex, we aimed to recruit 700 male and 700 female participants in each province. Assuming an average of 4 persons aged 5 years or older in each household, a total of 12 households in each of the 30 cluster was to be recruited in the survey. The total number of persons that would be recruited from the province was 1,806.

The sero-prevalence of children was about half that for older children, and in estimating the sample size for persons aged below 5 years, the following parameters were considered: a prevalence of 3.5%, desired precision or confidence interval (d) of +3.4%, and a design effect (DE) of 2 and an 80% response rate. The computed sample size was 282. Therefore, in each province 406 children would be recruited for the survey.

Included in the study were individuals aged 9 months or older who were found in a sampled household at the time of the study and were resident in the study site for at least seven days. Individuals who had received YF vaccination in the last ten years to the survey were also included in the survey. Excluded from the study were persons who were aged less than 9 months, or individuals regardless of age who resided in the study site for less than 7 days prior to the survey. Children under the age of 9 months were excluded based on the fact that at this age children could still carry maternal antibodies from exposed mothers which could pose the risk of false positive results.

The sample was drawn using a two-stage cluster sampling technique using probability proportional to size. A list of the standard enumeration areas (SEAs) in each province constituted the sampling frame. The line lists of the SEAs were provided by the Government's Central Statistics Office (CSO). The sampling was designed to achieve fairly good estimates at the provincial level of analysis, and not representing the subdivisions of the province.

STUDY VARIABLES

Dependent variable

A case with evidence of WNV exposure was defined as any individual aged 9 months or older whose blood sample was confirmed to have WNV exposure. WNV exposure status was positive if IgG or IgM antibodies were determined in the serum sample by laboratory testing and negative if the IgG or IgM antibodies were absent by laboratory testing.

Independent variables

The independent variables included demographic data: age, sex, occupation, education, roof type and use of mosquito preventive measures such as insecticide treated nets (ITNs) and indoor residual spray (IRS).

Laboratory procedures

Three to 5 millilitres of blood was collected by venepuncture into an EDTA vaccutainer tube and transported on cold chain to the local laboratories for serum separation and storage.

Subsequently serum samples were transported on cold chain and thereafter subjected to primary testing (YFV specific IgG and IgM) at the University of Teaching Hospital in Zambia virology unit and Institute Pasteur, Dakar, Senegal. All presumptive YFV-specific IgG and IgM samples were subjected to IgG and IgM antibodies testing against other flaviviruses known to cause haemorrhagic fever-like disease including WNV. The testing was carried out using IgG capture enzyme-linked immunosorbent assay (ELISA).

Data management and analysis

Data collected from the field were entered in an Epi-Info data entry screen that had consistency and range checks embedded in it. Further editing was conducted by running frequencies during the analysis stage. Epi data files were exported to SPSS for data analysis. The data was summarized to describe the occurrence of WNV exposed individuals in absolute numbers and percentage by place (residence, travel or work) and person (age, sex, occupation, education). Further analysis using logistic regression was conducted to determine independent factors associated with WNV sero-positivity. Unadjusted Odds ratios (OR) and adjusted odds ratios (AOR) together with their 95% confidence intervals (CI) were used to estimate magnitudes of associations.

Ethical considerations

Ethical clearance was sought from the Tropical Diseases Research Centre Research Ethics Committee, and ethical standards were adhered to throughout this study. Informed consent was sought from study participants. Guardians provided assent for the participation of the persons under the consenting age. They were asked to read or have read to them, understand and sign/thumbprint an informed consent form. Responsible adults in the household were identified to give proxy consent on behalf of minors.

OUR FINDINGS

A total of 1,824 respondents participated in the survey of which 55.2% were females. About half (48.0%) of all the participants (46.8% male and 49.3% females) attained primary school level of education. Of the participants, 30.3% (34.3% males and 27% females) attained higher level of education. Meanwhile the rates of being infected with WNV were 18.3% (19% males and 17.7% females, p=0.512). These results are shown in Table 1.

Table 1. Sample description Western province

Factors	Total	%	Male	%	Female	%
Age (years) [x^2 =7.27, p=0.122]						
<15	655	36.0	312	38.3	342	34.0
15-24	390	21.4	180	22.1	210	20.9
25-34	245	13.5	94	11.4	151	15.0
25-44	213	11.7	93	11.4	120	11.9
45+	318	17.5	136	16.7	182	18.1
Sex						
Male	815	44.8				
Female	1005	55.2				
Education [x^2=12.83, p<0.002]						
None	388	21.5	152	18.9	235	23.6
Primary	868	48.2	376	46.8	492	49.3
Secondary	546	30.3	276	34.3	270	27.1
College / University						
West Nile Infection [x^2=0.43, p=0.512]						
Positive	334	18.3	155	19.0	178	17.7
Negative	1490	91.7	660	81.0	827	82.3

Variables that were considered in the analysis were age, sex, education level, sleeping under a mosquito net, using IRS and travel to DRC and to Angola (Table 2). Those below the age of 15 years were 61% (AOR 0.39 95% CI [0.30-0.51]) less likely to be infected with WNV compared to those above 15 years of age. Participants who had attained primary level of education were 44% (AOR 1.44, 95% CI [1.22-1.70]) more likely to be infected by the virus than those who had attained secondary or higher levels of education. Travelling to Congo DRC was not associated with acquiring the infection but those who travelled to Angola were 78% (AOR, 1.78, 95% CI [1.25-2.55]) more likely to be infected with the virus than those who did not travel. Meanwhile gender, sleeping under a mosquito net and house with IRS were not associated with WNV infection.

Table 2. Factors associated with West Nile Virus infection in bivariate and multivariate analysis for Western province

Factor	OR	95% CI	AOR	95% CI
Age (years)				
<15	0.42	(0.33-0.53)	0.39	(0.30-0.51)
15-24	0.84	(0.66-1.07)	0.93	(0.72-1,19)
25-34	1.20	(0.92-1.56)	1.25	(0.96-1.63)
35-44	1.24	(0.94-1.64)	1.20	(0.91-1.59)
45+	1	1	1	1
Sex				
Male	1.05	(0.64-0.97)		
Female		1		
Education				
None	0.79	(0.64-0.97)	0.89	(0.71-1.13)
Primary	1.34	(1.14-1.57)	1.44	(1.22-1.70)
Secondary	1	1	1	1
College/University				
Slept under mosquito net				
Yes	1.05	(0.93-1.19)		
No	1	1		
House with IRS				
Yes	0.92	(0.77-1.09)		
No	1			1
Travelled to Angola				
Yes	2.14	(1.52-3.02)	1.78	(1.25-2.55)
No	1		1	

DISCUSSION

This study provides the first evidence of the circulation of WNV and correlates for the infection in Western province of Zambia. The study has indicated that 18.3% of the participants in the yellow fever risk assessment survey had antibodies to WNV. This result is consistent with results from surveys conducted worldwide although in some areas very high seroprevalence was discovered. In Italy, the study conducted in blood donors had lower rates which ranged from 3-33/1000 blood donors (13). The seroprevalence in USA varied across the country with rates ranging from 4.2% to 19.7%. Disease prevalence is dependent upon a wide range of risk factors, climate and the environment affecting the activities of the virus and the humans (2, 9,10). In Africa higher rates (60-74%) in Egypt, (3-65%) in Kenya and (13-24%) in South Africa, were reported as way back as the 1950s to 1970s (14,15).

Age, education and travelling to Angola were significance associated with WNV infection. Participants younger than 15 years old were less likely to be infected with the virus. Activities associated with older age such as working outside homes may increase chances of being exposed to the mosquito vector carrying the virus. A similar finding has been reported by Liu et al. (2) who found that persons above the age of 50 years were more at risk for the disease compared to those below the age of 50 years. An increase in prevalence of antibodies against with age may suggest endemic infection (16).

The finding that education was significantly associated with infection was not consistent. While persons with no formal education were equally likely to have the infection as those with secondary of higher levels of education, persons with primary level of education were more likely to be infected. When comparing persons with no formal education with those who had attained primary level of education, the finding in the current study contradicts that found by Gibney et al. (1) who indicated that those who did not attend school and were more often at home were more at risk of the disease than those who were often attending school. It is not clear what exposure factors persons who had attained primary level of education had to have increased risk of infection.

West Nile virus has been active in Angola (17). Movement of people across the border between Zambia and Angola whether by motor vehicle or foot may increase the risk of introducing dengue fever from endemic to non-endemic areas (18). However, the fact that there has been no report on the infection in Western province, it does not exclude the province from being an endemic area for West Nile infection. In conclusion, WNV infection is common in Western province, and interventions should be designed taking into account the correlates for WNV infection that had been identified in the current study.

ACKNOWLEDGMENTS

We are grateful to the interviewers for their dedicated work to successfully complete the survey. The survey could not have been successful without the cooperation of the participants and the virology laboratory staff both in Lusaka, Zambia and Dakar, Senegal for in testing samples. The survey was funded by the Ministry of Health [Zambia] and the World Health Organization.

REFERENCES

[1] Gibney KB, Colborn J, Baty S, Bunko Patterson AM, Sylvester T, Briggs G, et al. Modifiable risk factors for West Nile virus infection during an outbreak--Arizona, 2010. Am J Trop Med Hyg 2012;86:895-901.

[2] Liu A, Lee V, Galusha D, Slade MD, Diuk-Wasser M, Andreadis T, et al. Risk factors for human infection with West Nile Virus in Connecticut: a multi-year analysis. Int J Health Geogr 2009;8:67.

[3] Nash D, Mostashari F, Fine A, Miller J, O'Leary D, Murray K, et al. 1999 West Nile Outbreak Response Working Group. The outbreak of West Nile virus infection in the New York City area in 1999. N Engl J Med 2001;344:1807-14.

[4] LaBeaud AD, Kile JR, Kippes C, King CH, Mandalakas AM. Exposure to West Nile virus during the 2002 epidemic in Cuyahoga County, Ohio: a comparison of pediatric and adult behaviors. Public Health Rep 2007;122:356-61.

[5] Petersen LR, Carson PJ, Biggerstaff BJ, Custer B, Borchardt SM, Busch MP. Estimated cumulative incidence of West Nile virus infection in US adults, 1999-2010. Epidemiol Infect. 2013;141:591-5.

[6] Smithburn KC, Hughes TP, Burke AW, Paul JH. A Neurotropic Virus Isolated from the Blood of a Native of Uganda. Am J Trop Med 1940;20:471-2.

[7] Stiasny K, Aberle SW, Heinz FX. Retrospective identification of human cases of West Nile virus infection in Austria (2009 to 2010) by serological differentiation from Usutu and other flavivirus infections. Euro Surveill. 2013;18(43):pii=20614

[8] Schweitzer BK, Kramer WL, Sambol AR, Meza JL, Hinrichs SH, Iwen PC. Geographic factors contributing to a high seroprevalence of West Nile virus-specific antibodies in humans following an epidemic. Clin Vaccine Immunol 2006; 13(3):314-8.

[9] Brown HE, Childs JE, Diuk-Wasser MA, Fish D. Ecological factors associated with West Nile virus transmission, northeastern United States. Emerg Infect Dis 2008;14:1539-45.

[10] Gibbs SEJ, Wimberly MC, Madden M, Masour J, Yabsley MJ, Stallknecht DE. Factors affecting the geographic distribution of West Nile virus in Georgia, USA: 2002–2004. Vector Borne Zoonotic Dis 2006;6:73-82.

[11] Jentes ES, Poumerol G, Gershman MD, Hill DR, Lemarchand J, Lewis RF, et al. The revised global yellow fever risk map and recommendations for vaccination, 2010: consensus of the Informal WHO Working Group on Geographic Risk for Yellow Fever. Lancet Infect Dis 2011;11:622-32.

[12] Central Statistical Office. 2010 census of population and housing. National analytical report. Lusaka, Zambia: CSO, 2012.

[13] Pezzotti P, Piovesan C, Barzon L, Cusinato R, Cattai M, Pacenti M, et al. Prevalence of IgM and IgG antibodies to West Nile virus among blood donors in an affected area of north-eastern Italy, summer 2009. Euro Surveill 2011;16(10):pii=1981

[14] Darwish M A, Ibrahim AH. Survey for antibodies to arboviruses in Egyptian sera. I. West Nile virus antihemagglutinins in human and animal sera. Egypt Public Health Assoc 1971;46:61-70.

[15] Murgue B, Murri S, Triki H, Deubel V, Zeller HG. West Nile in the Mediterranean basin: 1950-2000. Ann N Y Acad Sci 2001;951:117-26.

[16] Fagbami AH, Monath TP, Fabiyi A. Dengue virus infections in Nigeria: a survey for antibodies in monkeys and humans. Trans R Soc Trop Med Hyg 1977;71:60–5.

[17] Kokernot RH, Casaca VMR, Weinbren MP, McIntosh BM. Survey for antibodies against arthropod-borne viruses in the sera of indigenous residents of Angola. *Trans R Soc Trop Med Hyg* 1965);59:563-70.

[18] Blackburn NK, Rawat R. Dengue fever imported from India: a report of 3 cases. S Afr Med J 1987;71:386-7.

In: Arbovirus
Editors: S. Siziya, M. L. Mazaba et al.
ISBN: 978-1-63463-601-8

Chapter 12

AEDES SPECIES MOSQUITO IN NORTH-WESTERN PROVINCE OF ZAMBIA: OBSERVATION DURING A YELLOW FEVER RISK ASSESSMENT SURVEY

Freddie Masaninga*[1,*]*, Mbanga Muleba*[2]*,
Osbert Namafente*[2]*, Peter Songolo*[1]*,
Idah Mweene-Ndumba*[1]*, Mazyanga L Mazaba*[1]*,
Mulakwa Kamuliwo*[3]*, Seter Siziya*[4,5]
and Olusegun A Babaniyi*[1]
[1]World Health Organization (WHO), Lusaka, Zambia,
[2]Tropical Diseases Research Centre, Ndola, Zambia,
[3]Ministry of Health, Zambia,
[4]School of Medicine, Copperbelt University, Ndola, Zambia,
[5]University of Lusaka, Lusaka, Zambia

Although records on mosquitoes belonging to *Aedes* date back to 1950s, there is paucity of knowledge on the distribution, species composition and bionomics of arthropod-borne vectors in Zambia. In 2013, during a yellow fever risk assessment survey conducted in North-Western province of Zambia, an entomological survey was conducted to

* Corresponding author: Freddie Masaninga, PhD, National Professional Officer, WHO Country Office, Lusaka, Zambia. E-mail: Masaningaf@who.int.

ascertain the availability, density and infectivity of yellow fever vectors in the province. We present information on *Aedes* species which was not identified into *Aedes (Stegomyia) aegypti, Aedes simpsoni*, or any other previously collected mosquitoes. *Aedes* species were collected in forested and peri-urban locations of North-Western province. Approximately 75% were classified as *Aedes (Finlaya) wellani*, while the rest were classified as *Aedes (Stegomyia) aegypti, Aedes (Stegomyia) africanus, Aedes (aedimorphus) mutilus* and *Aedes (aedimorphus) minutus*. Literature search showed that this is the first collection of *Aedes (Finlaya) wellani* in Zambia. Analysis of *Aedes* species (N=60) using the Polymerase Chain Reaction (PCR) for viral infection showed no viral activity. Observation of *Aedes (Finlaya) wellani* which has hitherto not been reported in Zambia indicates the importance of strengthened entomological surveillance in Zambia.

INTRODUCTION

Studies on *Aedes* species distribution, bionomics and species composition in Zambia are limited and systematic reports date back to 1950s. Mosquito vector studies have tended to focus on vectors of malaria (1,2). Malaria is ranked among the top ten common causes of illness in the country. In 2013, during a yellow fever risk assessment survey, an entomological survey was conducted to ascertain the availability, density and infectivity of yellow fever vectors in North-Western province of Zambia.

OUR STUDY

The study was conducted in North-Western province of Zambia in six districts, namely, Mwinilunga, Mufumbwe, Kabompo, Chavuma, Solwezi and Zambezi. North-Western province is located at 1,354 metres above sea level, latitude -13.0 and longitude 25.0 and has a population of 706,462. The province borders with Angola on the western side and the Democratic Republic of Congo on the northern side. Highest rainfall in the country, with annual rainfall of 1320 mm is recorded in this province. The mean minimum temperature in the dry cold month of June is 6.8°C and the mean maximum temperature in dry hot month October is30.6°C (3). The province is located within the Central African plateau.

Mosquito sampling

Sampling was conducted in April-May 2013, in the transition from wet to the drier month (3).

Larvae: Larval searches were conducted in rural, urban and peri-urban areas of the province. Both inside and outside houses were searched for larvae. The survey team covered at least 10 households per day. The term household meant one or more people who lived in the same dwelling and also shared meals or living accommodation.

Indoor inspection included flower-pots and water storage, whereas outside inspection included wells, discarded Clay-pots, discarded bottles and plastic containers; banana (*Musa sapientum*) leaf axils, discarded tyres and edges of water canals. The collected mosquito larvae were kept in larval bottles (Figure 1). Mosquito larval data included province, district, locality (urban or rural), house number (randomly allocated during sampling) and date of collection.

Adults: Adult mosquitoes were sampled by three research teams consisting of four persons per team. The following sampling methods were used to collect adult mosquitoes: backpack aspirators, aspiration using a mouth aspirator tube, CDC light trap and the Gravid Light traps. Mosquito collections were made inside and outside households in different ecological locations: rural, urban, forest and plains. Outdoor mosquitoes were captured using backpack aspirator, CDC light trap and Gravid light trap for collecting gravid (egg-laying) females to increase the chance for virus isolation. Sampling mosquitoes using back pack aspirator was conducted outdoor between 1600 and 1900 hours. Indoor adult resting mosquitoes were collected by various methods such as mouth aspirator tube using a torch to locate these resting sites and knockdown spray catch with pyrethroids insecticide in randomly selected dwellings which commenced at 0600 hours. All adult mosquitoes collected from the field were sorted and pooled by site of collection, sex and stored in liquid nitrogen to maintain mosquito morphological features

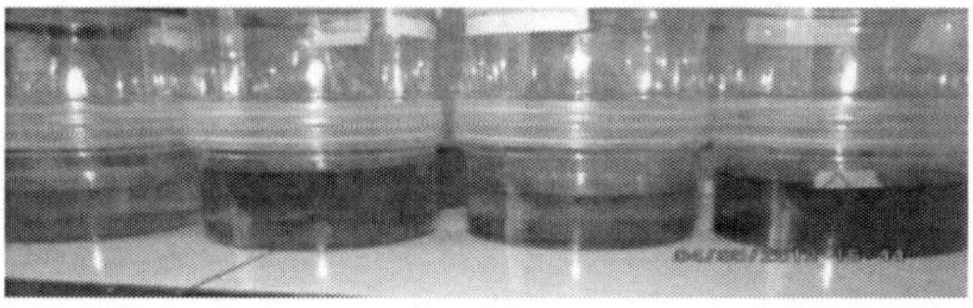

Figure 1. Mosquito Larvae kept for emerging into adult in TDRC, Ndola, Zambia.

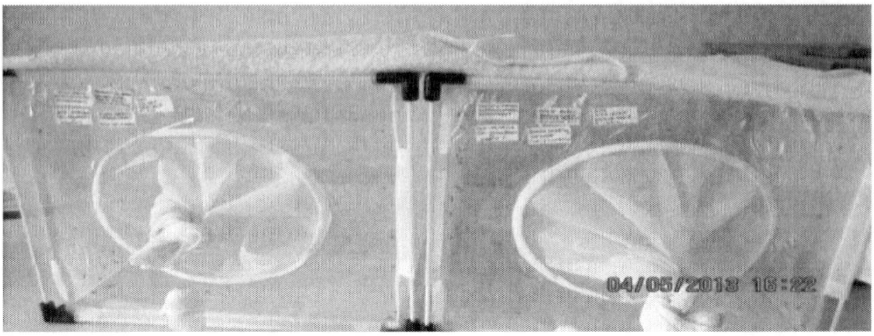

Figure 2. Field collected adult mosquitoes in cages transported to TDRC, Ndola, Zambia.

Mosquito larval rearing

Sampled mosquito larvae were transported to the Tropical Diseases Research Centre (TDRC) Insectary Laboratory in Ndola, Zambia, to rear them into the adult stage for species identification using entomological keys (5-7). At the TDRC Laboratory the larvae were fed on fish flakes Tetramin and maintained at relative humidity of 80±2% and temperature 23±2°C. Emerged adult mosquitoes were stored at -80˚C to preserve their viability.

Shipment, viral tests and vector species identification

Sixty adult *Aedes* species mosquitoes were airfreighted to Institute Pasteur in Dakar (IPD), Senegal to test for the presence of arthropod-borne viral activity in the *Aedes* specimen vector species by Reverse Transcriptase Polymerase Chain reaction (RT-PCR) technique and to identify and or validate the sub-sample species. In transit to IPD, the mosquito specimens were preserved at -80°C in dry ice to maintain DNA viability.

Ethical considerations

Each participant in the study had earlier been vaccinated against yellow fever virus and received prior chemoprophylaxis against malaria (4). The protocol was approved by the Tropical Diseases Research Centre Research Ethics Committee in Ndola, Zambia. Permission to access houses was sought from heads of houses.

OUR FINDINGS

Out of a total of 453 *adult Aedes* species of mosquitoes collected from rural, urban, peri-urban and forest locations, the majority (75.47%) were classified as *Aedes (Finlaya) wellani* (Figures 3 and 4).

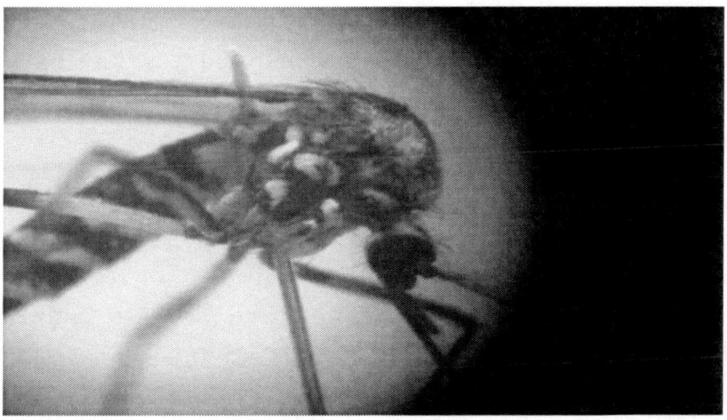

Figure 3. Field collected adult Aedes (Finlaya) Wellani side view.

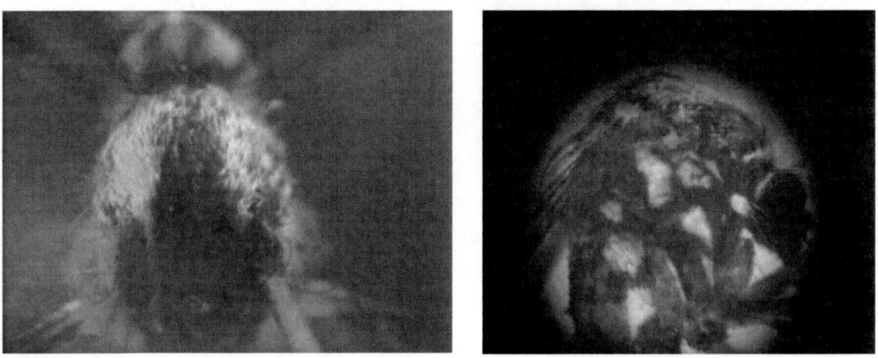

Figure 4. Dorsal head view of Aedes (Finalaya) wellani; collected from Ikelenge, Zambezi district Zambia.

Aedes (Finlaya) wellani were collected from Ikelenge, situated near the source of the river Zambezi in the Zambezi district of Zambia. The other Aedes species that were collected are *Aedes (Stegomyia) aegypti, Aedes (Stegomyia) africanus, Aedes (aedimorphus) mutilus* and *Aedes (aedimorphus) minutus.*

None of the 60 female *Aedes* species of *Aedes (stegomia) aegypti*, *Aedes (stegomyia) africanus, Aedes (aedimorphus) minutus*, *Aedes (aedimorphus) mutilus* and *Aedes (Finlaya) wellmani* were positive for the yellow fever virus.

DISCUSSION

This study has identified *Aedes* mosquitoes collected from Ikelenge, Zambezi district, which did not belong to the species reported by the previous investigators (8). Independent verification at a WHO accredited, collaboration centre of the mosquito specimens, identified it as *Aedes (Finlaya) wellani.* To our knowledge this is the first report of this *Aedes* species at Ikelenge, Zambezi district in Zambia.

More studies should be conducted to study the behaviour, spatial and geographical distribution of this mosquito in North-Western province and other provinces in Zambia to gain more accurate understanding on the possible role of *Aedes (Finlaya) wellani* in the transmission of arboviruses in Zambia.

Entomological studies on mosquito vector distribution are critical given the increasingly importance of new emerging arthropod-borne infections such as Zika, Dengue and reports of expansion through increased global trade and climatic changes which are being reported in Africa, Asia and other regions (9). Strengthening entomological surveillance becomes imperative in Zambia in order to provide accurate data base for evidenced-based vector control decisions.

In conclusion, collection of *Aedes (Finlaya) wellani* during a yellow fever risk assessment survey in Zambia underpins the increasing need to maintain a strong entomological surveillance in-country for guiding rational vector control programs.

REFERENCES

[1] Littrell M, Miller JM, Ndhlovu M, Hamainza B, Hawela M, Kamuliwo M, et al. Documenting malaria case management coverage in Zambia: a systems effectiveness Approach. Malar J 2013;12:371.

[2] Masaninga F, Chanda E, Chanda-Kapata P, Hamainza B, Masendu HT, Kamuliwo M, et al. Review of the malaria epidemiology and trends in Zambia. Asian Pac J Trop Biomed 2013;3:89-94.

[3] North-Western province, Zambia 2010. Accessed 2014 August 27. URL: http://1worldmap.com/Zambia/North-Western-Province.

[4] WHO. Meeting of the Strategic Advisory Group of Experts on immunization, April 2013 – Conclusions and Recommendations. Weekly Epidemiol Record 2013;88:201–16.

[5] Gillies MT and Coetzee M. A supplement to the Anophelinae of Africa south of the Sahara (Afrotropical Region). Johannesburg: Publications of the South African Institute for Medical Research, 1987.

[6] Rueda ML. Pictorial keys for the identification of mosquitoes (Diptera: Culicidae) associated with Dengue Virus Transmission. Auckland, New Zealand: Magnolia Press, 2004:14-20.

[7] Yiau-Min H. A pictorial key for the identification of the subfamilies of Culicidae, genera of Culicinae, and subgenera of Aedes mosquitoes of the Afrotropical region (Diptera: Culicidae). Proceedings of the Entomological Society of Washington 2001;103:1-53.

[8] Robinson GG. A note on mosquitoes and yellow fever in Northern Rhodesia. East Afr Med J 1950;27:284-8.

[9] Dash AP, Bhatia R, Sunyoto T, Mourya DT. Emerging and re-emerging arboviral diseases in South East Asia. J Vector Borne Dis 2013;50:77-84.

SECTION TWO: ACKNOWLEDGMENTS

In: Arbovirus
Editors: S. Siziya, M. L. Mazaba et al.
ISBN: 978-1-63463-601-8

Chapter 13

About the Editors

Seter Siziya, BA(Ed), MSc, PhD, CStat, CSci, FRSS, born in Lusaka, Zambia, is a professor of medical biostatistics with the Copperbelt University in the School of Medicine, Ndola Central Hospital in Zambia. He was recognized as one of the Hot 100 authors worldwide for the BioMed Central Journals in 2007; awarded a certificate of achievement by the Copperbelt University for outstanding achievement in research at the Copperbelt University School of Medicine in 2012; Received a Vice-Chancellor's award for excellence for the years in 2013 at the Copperbelt University; and received a meritorious award for excellence in research and academic development from the Zambia Medical Association in 2013. He previously worked for the Tropical Diseases Research Centre, Ndola, Zambia; University of Zimbabwe and the University of Zambia. He has been teaching biostatistics, epidemiology and research methods to both undergraduate and postgraduate students in the universities he has worked in. He has been a reviewer, editorial member and associate editor for international journals. He has published numerous papers on tobacco smoking, HIV, Integrated management of childhood illnesses, immunization, measles, non-communicable diseases, suicide, bullying, alcohol and occupational health. E-mail: ssiziya@gmail.com

Mazyanga L Mazaba, BSc, MSc, graduated from the University of Zambia, School of Medicine. She specialises in the areas of virology and public health (vaccines and preventable diseases). She is currently a laboratory scientist and data manager with the World Health Organization under the Expanded Program on Immunisation (EPI), particularly, polio, measles, rubella, influenza, rota virus and yellow fever surveillance and involved in laboratory diagnosis and training laboratory and surveillance personnel in sample collection and management. She has vast experience in immunology, virology, various diagnostic methods and data management. She has published in a variety of peer reviewed journals and presented papers at international and national conferences in the field of virology and epidemiology. She is now working in the field of epidemiology as she pursues a DSc in epidemiology. E-mail: liwewem@who.int

Joav Merrick, MD, MMedSci, DMSc, born and educated in Denmark is professor of pediatrics, child health and human development, Division of Pediatrics, Hadassah Hebrew University Medical Center, Mt Scopus Campus, Jerusalem, Israel and Kentucky Children's Hospital, University of Kentucky, Lexington, Kentucky United States and professor of public health at the Center for Healthy Development, School of Public Health, Georgia State University, Atlanta, United States, the medical director of the Health Services, Division for Intellectual and Developmental Disabilities, Ministry of Social Affairs and Social Services, Jerusalem, the founder and director of the National Institute of Child Health and Human Development in Israel. Numerous publications in the field of pediatrics, child health and human development, rehabilitation, intellectual disability, disability, health, welfare, abuse, advocacy, quality of life and prevention. Received the Peter Sabroe Child Award for outstanding work on behalf of Danish Children in 1985 and the International LEGO-Prize ("The Children's Nobel Prize") for an extraordinary contribution towards improvement in child welfare and well-being in 1987. E-mail: jmerrick@zahav.net.il

In: Arbovirus
Editors: S. Siziya, M. L. Mazaba et al.
ISBN: 978-1-63463-601-8

Chapter 14

About the National Institute of Child Health and Human Development in Israel

The National Institute of Child Health and Human Development (NICHD) in Israel was established in 1998 as a virtual institute under the auspicies of the Medical Director, Ministry of Social Affairs and Social Services in order to function as the research arm for the Office of the Medical Director. In 1998 the National Council for Child Health and Pediatrics, Ministry of Health and in 1999 the Director General and Deputy Director General of the Ministry of Health endorsed the establishment of the NICHD.

Mission

The mission of a National Institute for Child Health and Human Development in Israel is to provide an academic focal point for the scholarly interdisciplinary study of child life, health, public health, welfare, disability, rehabilitation, intellectual disability and related aspects of human development. This mission includes research, teaching, clinical work, information and public service activities in the field of child health and human development.

Service and academic activities

Over the years many activities became focused in the south of Israel due to collaboration with various professionals at the Faculty of Health Sciences (FOHS) at the Ben Gurion University of the Negev (BGU). Since 2000 an affiliation with the Zusman Child Development Center at the Pediatric Division of Soroka University Medical Center has resulted in collaboration around the establishment of the Down Syndrome Clinic at that center. In 2002 a full course on "Disability" was established at the Recanati School for Allied Professions in the Community, FOHS, BGU and in 2005 collaboration was started with the Primary Care Unit of the faculty and disability became part of the master of public health course on "Children and society". In the academic year 2005-2006 a one semester course on "Aging with disability" was started as part of the master of science program in gerontology in our collaboration with the Center for Multidisciplinary Research in Aging. In 2010 collaborations with the Division of Pediatrics, Hadassah Hebrew University Medical Center, Jerusalem, Israel around the National Down Syndrome Center and teaching students and residents about intellectual and developmental disabilities as part of their training at this campus.

Research activities

The affiliated staff have over the years published work from projects and research activities in this national and international collaboration. In the year 2000 the International Journal of Adolescent Medicine and Health and in 2005 the International Journal on Disability and Human Development of De Gruyter Publishing House (Berlin and New York) were affiliated with the National Institute of Child Health and Human Development. From 2008 also the International Journal of Child Health and Human Development (Nova Science, New York), the International Journal of Child and Adolescent Health (Nova Science) and the Journal of Pain Management (Nova Science) affiliated and from 2009 the International Public Health Journal (Nova Science) and Journal of Alternative Medicine Research (Nova Science). All peer-reviewed international journals.

NATIONAL COLLABORATIONS

Nationally the NICHD works in collaboration with the Faculty of Health Sciences, Ben Gurion University of the Negev; Department of Physical Therapy, Sackler School of Medicine, Tel Aviv University; Autism Center, Assaf HaRofeh Medical Center; National Rett and PKU Centers at Chaim Sheba Medical Center, Tel HaShomer; Department of Physiotherapy, Haifa University; Department of Education, Bar Ilan University, Ramat Gan, Faculty of Social Sciences and Health Sciences; College of Judea and Samaria in Ariel and in 2011 affiliation with Center for Pediatric Chronic Diseases and National Center for Down Syndrome, Department of Pediatrics, Hadassah Hebrew University Medical Center, Mount Scopus Campus, Jerusalem.

INTERNATIONAL COLLABORATIONS

Internationally with the Department of Disability and Human Development, College of Applied Health Sciences, University of Illinois at Chicago; Strong Center for Developmental Disabilities, Golisano Children's Hospital at Strong, University of Rochester School of Medicine and Dentistry, New York; Centre on Intellectual Disabilities, University of Albany, New York; Centre for Chronic Disease Prevention and Control, Health Canada, Ottawa; Chandler Medical Center and Children's Hospital, Kentucky Children's Hospital, Section of Adolescent Medicine, University of Kentucky, Lexington; Chronic Disease Prevention and Control Research Center, Baylor College of Medicine, Houston, Texas; Division of Neuroscience, Department of Psychiatry, Columbia University, New York; Institute for the Study of Disadvantage and Disability, Atlanta; Center for Autism and Related Disorders, Department Psychiatry, Children's Hospital Boston, Boston; Department of Pediatric and Adolescent Medicine, Western Michigan University Homer Stryker MD School of Medicine, Kalamazoo, Michigan, United States; Department of Paediatrics, Child Health and Adolescent Medicine, Children's Hospital at Westmead, Westmead, Australia; International Centre for the Study of Occupational and Mental Health, Düsseldorf, Germany; Centre for Advanced Studies in Nursing, Department of General Practice and Primary Care, University of Aberdeen, Aberdeen, United Kingdom; Quality of Life Research Center, Copenhagen, Denmark; Nordic School of Public Health, Gottenburg, Sweden, Scandinavian Institute of Quality of Working Life, Oslo, Norway;

The Department of Applied Social Sciences (APSS) of The Hong Kong Polytechnic University Hong Kong.

TARGETS

Our focus is on research, international collaborations, clinical work, teaching and policy in health, disability and human development and to establish the NICHD as a permanent institute at one of the residential care centers for persons with intellectual disability in Israel in order to conduct model research and together with the four university schools of public health/medicine in Israel establish a national master and doctoral program in disability and human development at the institute to secure the next generation of professionals working in this often non-prestigious/low-status field of work.

CONTACT

Joav Merrick, MD, MMedSci, DMSc
Professor of Pediatrics, Child Health and Human Development
Medical Director, Health Services,
Division for Intellectual and Developmental Disabilities,
Ministry of Social Affairs and Social Services,
POB 1260, IL-91012 Jerusalem, Israel.
E-mail: jmerrick@zahav.net.il

In: Arbovirus ISBN: 978-1-63463-601-8
Editors: S. Siziya, M. L. Mazaba et al.

Chapter 15

About the Book Series "Public Health: Practices, Methods and Policies"

Public health is a book series with publications from a multidisciplinary group of researchers, practitioners and clinicians for an international professional forum interested in the broad spectrum of public health issues. Books already published:

- Rubin IL, Merrick J, eds. Environment and public health: Environmental health, law and international perspectives. New York: Nova Science, 2014.
- Shek DTL, Siu AMH, Merrick J, eds. Tomorrow's leaders: Service leadership and holistic development in Chinese university students. New York: Nova Science, 2015.

Contact

Professor Joav Merrick, MD, MMedSci, DMSc
Medical Director, Health Services
Division for Intellectual and Developmental Disabailities
Ministry of Social Affairs and Social Services
POBox 1260, IL-91012 Jerusalem, Israel
E-mail: jmerrick@zahav.net.il

SECTION THREE: INDEX

INDEX

E

F

G

L

M

N

O

P

Q

R

S

T

U

V

W

Z